A quick guide™ to clinical trials

"for people who may not know it all"

EDITED BY:

Drs. Madhu Davies and Faiz Kermani

April 2008

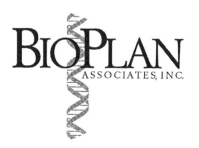

BioPlan Associates, Inc.

Rockville, MD

BioPlan Associates, Inc.
2275 Research Blvd, Suite 500
Rockville MD 20850 USA
301-921-5979
www.bioplanassociates.com

For information on special discounts or permissions contact BioPlan Associates, Inc. at 301-921-5979, or info@bioplanassociates.com

Production: E.S. Illustration & Design, Inc.
Text and Cover Design: E.S. Illustration & Design, Inc.

ISBN 978-1-934106-08-2
Second Printing 2010

BOOK REVIEWS

"Clinical trials are the single most resource-intensive investment in bringing a drug to market. Davies and Kermani have created a primer that should be essential reading for any healthcare professional and life scientist who want to understand this complex, billion-dollar process."

– Jane Chin, Ph.D. President, Medical Science Liaison Institute

"This book provides a broad overview of the complex issues involved in the design, conduct and oversight of clinical trials. The authors bring a 'hands-on' expertise and diversity of perspectives to the book. Clearly and simply written, the book will be especially useful for readers who are new to clinical trials regardless of their role, or for experienced readers who want to refresh their knowledge of aspects to which they are less frequently exposed."

– Robert "Skip" Nelson, MD PhD, Pediatric Ethicist,
Office of Pediatric Therapeutics, US Food and Drug Administration

"As a job recruiter to this industry, I would strongly urge each and every candidate considering a career in clinical research to read this book. Armed with this knowledge and wisdom, they will have an advantage over others who have not read it."

– Austen Yapp, Founder & Director, Jobs.LeadDiscovery Ltd

"An excellent resource. Chapters 5 and 6 will be invaluable for new starters working in pharma or contract research. Given the current surge in recruitment, this may assist with the challenge of training to GCP standards. Chapter 11 on technology will introduce or explain the rise in the use of electronic data solutions and will raise the issue of management of the vendors, while Chapter 12 will illustrate ways of finding patients and the challenges of retaining them in trials."

– Sian Hingston, Head of Clinical Resourcing,
Global Clinical Operations Europe, GSK.

"This book covers the bases for anyone interested in clinical trials."

– Professor John Staniforth, CSO, PharmaKodex Ltd, UK

"An excellent resource to demystify the world of clinical trials."

– Rod Richards, CEO PharmaKodex Ltd, UK

"An excellent resource!"

– Anil Vaidya, CEO, Iatro Medical Systems

"As clinical trials become more complex, here's a book that still manages to keep the subject simple."

– Andrea Palluch, Director, Inpharmedia

"As a medical writer I found that this book provided an excellent overview of my specialization, but it also allowed me insight into other areas of clinical trials."

– Leigh van Wyk, Medical Writer

"Whether you represent the sponsor or the CRO, this book is a must-read for anyone involved in understanding the latest developments in the clinical trial process."

– Ronald R. Baker, Director of Business Development - North America, SGS Life Science Services

"This book is a great teaching tool. Some of the chapters are priceless (such as "Clinical Trials and the Patient"), while others provide deep content on a multitude of subjects."

– Suzanne M. Sensabaugh, MS, MBA, Vice President Biopharmaceutical Development, MDS Pharma Services

"An excellent book to add to your clinical trials library. There are books that deal with the theoretical aspects, and "cookbooks" that try to tell you exactly what to do. This book is special in that it adds a new element; it also tells you about clinical trials in a very practical way – what the job is about. This one adds a new, refreshing perspective and definitely belongs on your bookshelf."

– Steven E. Linberg, Ph.D., Managing Director, Chiesi Pharmaceuticals Inc.

Acknowledgment

This book was inspired by the enthusiasm about clinical trials shown by the many new recruits to the pharmaceutical industry we have met at scientific meetings we have attended over the years. It is also the book Madhu would have liked to have read when she joined the industry in 1993.

The book would not have been possible without the corresponding commitment shown by the authors, all of whom are well established experts in their fields and yet retain the ability to communicate on a level accessible to non-expert readers. And the imagination of the publisher, Eric Langer. We thank you all.

Both of us are particularly grateful to our own long suffering families who have provided cheerful support (and many cups of tea) during the gestation of this book.

For Miranda, Julia and Isis: keep asking those tricky questions; retain that curiosity!

Madhu Davies and Faiz Kermani

Contents

About the contributors

✳ **Dr. Bill Byrom** joined the Pharmaceutical industry in 1991 after completing a Ph.D. in disease control simulation at Strathclyde University, and has worked in a number of roles within Statistics, Clinical Development and International Marketing. At ClinPhone, Bill is Vice President of Product Strategy and Marketing with responsibilities for new areas of technology application within clinical trials and healthcare. Bill is the author of over 50 published articles and chapters in professional journals and publications.

✳ **Dr. Madhu Davies** qualified in medicine in the United Kingdom in 1987. Following six years in the clinic in general medical specialties and general practice, she joined the pharmaceutical industry looking for a public health challenge. Since that time she has enjoyed a variety of roles in medical affairs, clinical development, drug safety and regulatory affairs which has provided a broad foundation and experience. She is a Fellow of the Faculty of Pharmaceutical Medicine. Currently working as a consultant in pharmaceutical medicine, she is also editor of "Pharmaceutical Physician," the eponymously titled journal of the British Association of Pharmaceutical Physicians, an examiner for the Diploma in Pharmaceutical Medicine of the Royal College of Physicians (UK) and a senior specialty advisor for specialist training in pharmaceutical medicine. She has previously co-edited the book "Patient Compliance: Sweetening the Pill" with Dr. Faiz Kermani and published articles in professional journals.

✳ **Dr. Ignazio di Giovanna** holds a BSc in Physiology and Ph.D. in Biophysics from the University of London and joined the Pharmaceutical industry in 1986, since which he's worked both within the pharma and CRO settings. Ignazio has been Managing Director of Campbell Charles Associates 2000 Ltd since 1998, a CRO which provides clinical trial monitoring and management services. Following a period on the Institute of the Clinical Research board of directors, he was elected Chairman. Ignazio is currently President of Clinical Contract Research Association and a member of the Biotechnology & Pharmaceuticals Sector Advisory Group (Bpsag), to advise and influence UKTI on trade and investment matters, with a view to increasing both for the UK economy. Ignazio has also worked on a number of other industry related initiatives with the ABPI, NHS, R&D Forums and UKCRN.

✳ **Ms. Sue Green** has worked in global regulatory affairs for over 17 years. Having worked as a Regulatory Director for a number of pharmaceutical companies, she established her own consultancy company, Shore Limited with her business partner Heather Ninnes in April 2003. Shore provides regulatory support and strategic advice for all areas of drug development, registration and life-cycle management. More information on Sue and Shore Limited can be found on the company web-site www.shore.ltd.uk.

✳ **Dr. Felix Khin-Maung-Gyi** founded Chesapeake Research Review in 1993 and has managed its growth since the company's inception. Dr. Gyi is a recognized leader in human subject protection both in the US and abroad. In 2003, Dr. Gyi was appointed to the U.S. Secretary of Health and Human Services' Human Research Protections Advisory Committee (SACHRP) and served as a charter member until the end of his term in 2006. He currently Co-Chairs a subcommittee of SACHRP designated to review the interpretations and impact of regulations on the burdens and efficiencies of human research protections. Working with various international government agencies, he has advised on and conducted research ethics and GCP education programs in countries including India, Japan, Taiwan, Myanmar (Burma), Egypt, England, and Russia. Dr. Gyi received the Doctor of Pharmacy degree from Duquesne University; and the MBA (Executive Program) from Loyola (MD) College. He has completed Clinical Pharmacy residencies in both pediatric and adult medicine and postgraduate studies in bioethics, drug development, regulations and medical research. His undergraduate work in Pharmacy from the University of Maryland included a concentration in Microbiology.

✳ **Dr. Gareth Hayes** has over twenty-seven years industry experience behind him and continues to be at the forefront of our industry's training needs and regularly contributes articles to the journal CRfocus on the subject, e.g. Formulating Training Strategies, May 2004; Training Needs Analysis and Evaluation, November 2004; Championing Europe November 2005; Inspecting Training Records, February 2006. Gareth is a steering committee member of the Institute of Clinical Research Trainers' Forum.

✳ **Dr. Todd Johnson** brings 18 years' experience in life science research to his current position as Senior Vice President, Strategy and Corporate Development at MDS Pharma Services, a leading global contract research organization. In this role, he leads development of MDS's strategies to approach the drug development market, as well as the company's acquisitions and strategic partnerships. Prior to MDS, Todd spent five years with McKinsey & Company leading strategic consulting engagements at major pharmaceutical and biotech firms. Before McKinsey, he was Founder and CEO of Tangerine Technologies, a Philadelphia-based provider of drug discovery software. Before Tangerine, he spent time as a researcher at the Dana-Farber Cancer Institute, Harvard University, the University of Pennsylvania, and at the National Institutes of Health. Educated at Oxford University and the University of Pennsylvania, Todd holds an MBA from the Wharton School, an MD from Penn's Medical School, a BA in Neurobiology from Penn's College of Arts and Sciences' honors program, and an ABA from Oxford's St. Catherine's College.

✳ **Dr. Suzanne Junod** received her M.A. and Ph.D. from Emory University in the history of medicine. She came to the FDA as a historian in 1984. In 1994-5, she served as FDA liaison and historical consultant for President Clinton's Advisory Committee on Human Radiation Experiments (ACHRE). She is on the Editorial Board of the Journal of the History of Medicine and Allied Sciences and has written the "History Corner"-- a bimonthly column for the Food and Drug Law Institute's *Update* publication for the past decade. Her publications are wide-ranging in the history of medicine and public health, including women's health, history of food additive regulation, as well as food and drug legal, scientific, and regulatory issues. She has received several professional awards for her writing.

✳ **Dr. Faiz Kermani** has several years experience in both academia and the pharmaceutical industry. He has worked in pharmaceutical R&D, pricing and reimbursement, marketing and medical communications. He holds a Ph.D. in Immunopharmacology from St. Thomas' Hospital, London and a First Class Honors degree in Pharmacology with Toxicology from King's College, London. He has written extensively on international clinical trial issues. In March 2006, he was a delegate on the UK Government's Trade and Investment Biotech Scoping Mission to China and authored the clinical trials section of the subsequent report.

✳ **Ms. Liz Langley** graduated from Surrey University in 1978 with a BSc in Biochemistry (Medical), thus really trained to be a Clinical Chemist. However, in the careers office one day, she noticed the pharmaceutical industry as a career option and has been in and around it ever since. Having learned the rigors of selling at Merck, she joined the company's Medical Department and then followed a varied career path through clinical research, new product development, regional sales management and marketing. Liz has worked with the British Association of Pharmaceutical Physicians (BrAPP) since 1992 and is involved with the training, education and development of pharmaceutical physicians. She is also managing director of LHA Ltd.

✳ **Dr. Jim McClurg** has received alumni achievement awards from Nebraska Wesleyan and the University of Nebraska, has published a number of scientific articles, and holds a US patent in the field of laboratory testing. Prior to joining the CRO industry in 1976, Dr. McClurg served on the biochemistry faculty of the University of Nebraska Medical Center. He received his Ph.D. in Biochemistry from the University of Nebraska Medical Center, and holds a BS in Biology from Nebraska Wesleyan University. Jim serves as Senior Vice President and Chief Scientific Officer and leads the Strategic Client Relationship Team at MDS Pharma Services. This group develops and initiates new ways to do business with customers around the world, based on new business models, technology-enriched relationships, and the breadth and flexibility of MDS global services.

✳ **Ms. Lisa Nash** completed a BSc (Hons) in Chemistry from University College London in 1993 and went on to study for a Post Graduate Certificate in Education in Science at Homerton College, Cambridge. In 1994 she embarked on a career in teaching secondary school Science and later Mathematics. During 1997 she decided a career change was needed and discovered Data Management, quite accidentally. Since 1997 she has have worked as a contract Clinical Data Coordinator before joining the former SmithKline Beecham which became GlaxoSmithKline. Currently, she is a Therapeutic Programme Manager within Clinical Data Management. Much of her data management experience gathered over the last decade has been within the Infectious Diseases therapy area, in particular supporting a number of tropical disease trials in the developing world.

✳ **Ms. Cathy O'Brien** is a chartered statistician with over 20 years experience, the last 18 of which have been within the pharmaceutical industry. She graduated from London University in 1985 with a degree in Biology and Mathematics and started work as a statistician in horticultural research. Having worked for both a CRO and a pharmaceutical company, Cathy obtained an MSc in Medical Statistics from Leicester University. She is currently working as a statistical consultant through her own business.

✳ **Ms. Jan Robinson** obtained a BSc in Biological Sciences and then qualified as a nurse spending 11 years nursing in both hospital and community settings eventually specializing in intensive care. Her pharmaceutical career encompasses 9 years in the drug delivery arena, 4 years in medical devices and most recently 4 years in biologics at Cambridge Antibody Technology/Astra Zeneca in various project management roles covering all phases of development and a wide range of therapeutic areas. In October 2006 she joined the newly formed PharmaKodex Ltd, a UK based speciality pharmaceutical company, spun out of Unilever and Vectura. As Director of Clinical Operations she has responsibility for the strategic and operational delivery of clinical programs outsourcing all functions in a virtual environment. Jan was a founder member of and currently chairs the Institute of Clinical Research special interest group in Project Management.

✳ **Mr. David B. Stein**, has worked in Pharmaceutical technologies for over twenty years in a variety of roles. He has established the Data Management department for a mid-sized CRO, founded a start-up company providing mobile patient-reported outcomes and has created software for pharmaceutical post-marketing applications used in several countries. At ClinPhone, David is Vice President of Product Management with responsibilities for the company's portfolio of products and new areas of technology application within clinical trials and healthcare.

❋ **Ms. Fiona Swain** has 15 years' experience as a medical writer in the pharmaceutical industry. After studying for a BSc (Hons) in Pharmacology at Glasgow University, she gained accreditation from the American Medical Writers Association and is a member of the European Medical Writers Association. She has worked for a pharmaceutical company, a clinical research organization and as a freelance writer. Her main areas of expertise are in reporting clinical trials and writing summary documents for new drug license applications in America and Europe. Other documents she has written include clinical trial protocols, case report forms, investigator brochures, patient information leaflets, literature reviews, conference posters and training manuals.

❋ **Dr. Graham Wylie** is Chief Executive Officer of the Medical Research Network Ltd, an affiliate company of Healthcare at Home. Graham has 17 years experience in clinical trials, starting with 10 years at Pfizer in Clinical Development and Corporate HQ, with roles ranging from project management of trials to global implementation of standard trial processes and IT tools. He then joined Parexel International in 1999 as Medical Director for Northern Europe, progressing to Vice President of Account Management for Europe by 2003. In 2005 he joined Healthcare at Home to develop their clinical trials activities into a full business unit, known as 'The Medical Research Network,' spinning the division off as a separate company in 2006. The MRN provides Site Support, placing nurses in research sites; Home Trial Support, with nurses visiting patients in their own home for some trial visits and other services designed to directly address the needs of the UK research academic and pharmaceutical community.

Introduction

A quick guide to clinical trials:
"a book for people who may not know it all"
Drs. Madhu Davies and Faiz Kermani

What's in it for me: Why should I read this book?

Appropriately designed and executed clinical trials are at the heart of the successful development of new medicines for patients. Like any other specialized area, clinical trials has a vocabulary and jargon all its own and the processes involved are highly standardized for ethical, practical and regulatory reasons. No matter. With a little help from a friend, most people can get a grip on the topic in sufficient detail to understand in general terms what people are talking about. This book is that friend.

How we got to where we are is very important. The first part of this book provides a helicopter view of the clinical trials process with Chapter 1 explaining why we do what we do as a broad structure into which the later 'process' chapters will fit. The second chapter reviews the history of clinical trials *per se* and the evolving ethical and regulatory considerations (i.e., how we got to where we are). Complementing these two chapters is the commercial perspective: the imperative for moving forward.

Armed with these three chapters as background, the succeeding 'nuts and bolts' process chapters will fall into place. You will be able to see exactly how any given discipline fits in and plays its part in delivering the overall clinical trial program. For make no mistake, the successful design, execution and delivery of an effective clinical trial program relies on excellent cooperation, understanding and respect within an often widely dispersed multi-disciplinary team.

Faiz and I specifically set out to ask experienced clinical researchers from all the relevant disciplines to write succinct and straightforward chapters which would explain what their role is and how this fits into a very exciting big picture, overall. How does each group contribute to the team's success? The chapters are designed to be jargon-lite but yet, detailed enough to provide the framework onto which you, the reader, can attach that jargon when you are good and ready.

In addition, we felt it was very important to acknowledge the role of the patient because without their participation no clinical trial would proceed. Frequently, it is the enthusiasm and dedication of patients that keep clinical trials on track. There is currently a great need for a better public support of clinical trials, but this can only happen if both patients and clinical trial researchers fully engage with each other. Many clinical researchers are highly experienced in the operational and regulatory aspects of trials, but how many of them have actually become involved as a patient? The answer is probably very few! In combination with the other contributions, Chapter 13 helps fill this 'gap' as it is written by someone who has both worked on clinical trials and yet also participated as a patient.

We have tried to present these chapters in a logical way so that the flow of the clinical trials process is also apparent. This is rather artificial, as it will be clear to those who read the book straight through, that many activities happen in parallel and that while there is relatively little 'down time' for any specific group, there are often times of frenzied activity! Each chapter also stands alone as a 'quick dip' foundation or refresher.

Everyone involved in clinical trials finds it demanding to keep up-to-date with current developments in the field. Therefore, as a final aspect to the book we have tried to explore what the future of clinical trials might be. There are numerous factors that have shaped clinical trials until now and far more that will influence their development in the future. We can only guess at what the future of clinical trials might be, but one certainty is that we will continue to rely on them for the development of new medicines.

So why should you read this book? Because we believe you will come away with a really good basic grasp of the excitement of the clinical trials process, its drivers, checks and balances, and how you may even be able to contribute in a wide variety of ways.

Madhu Davies and Faiz Kermani
April 2008

Chapter 1

Why do we do clinical trials?

Dr. Graham Wylie, CEO Medical Research Network Ltd.

All clinical trials are unique, designed to answer a specific question.

Introduction

Clinical trials are a tool used to provide knowledge about a drug to physicians and governments, and to other organizations controlling the use of medicines in society. Some basic principles govern how clinical trials are designed:

1. Giving anyone an untried medication is a considerable risk.

2. Clinical trials in humans build slowly as experience is gained about a new drug.

3. All trials conform to a detailed and voluminous set of regulatory standards.

These are relatively self-explanatory and we will not deal with them in detail. However, two further concepts are worthy of detailed consideration:

4. Trials are scientific experiments – we are asking questions to which we do not know the answers.

5. Measuring medical outcomes is complex and often requires a mix of objective measurements (clearly defined and measurable) and subjective measurements (based on opinion and experience).

> Clinical trials are a tool used to provide knowledge about a drug to physicians and governments, and to other organizations controlling the use of medicines in society.

Before exploring these last two concepts, this chapter first covers the early research that is conducted before trials can even take place. We then provide a description of the most common types of clinical trials, and the details of how these trials are scientifically constructed or designed (essentially those elements that make each trial unique), and the elements in trials driven by regulatory and other requirements (essentially those elements that are common to all trials). The chapter finishes by looking at weaknesses in clinical trial design and future developments that might address these weaknesses.

This chapter provides a basic framework to help understand most trials the reader is likely to come across, and to set the scene for the subsequent chapters which describe the different functions at pharmaceutical companies needed to ensure trials take place as required.

For the purposes of this book, the trials described are those used to develop a new drug for the market place and ultimately to support it through its commercial life. Many other types of trial exist, studying other therapies, the behavior of the underlying condition, the basic pathological mechanisms involved in disease, etc. The concepts for these trials are the similar, so although we do not cover them in detail, the reader should be able to understand these trials, as well.

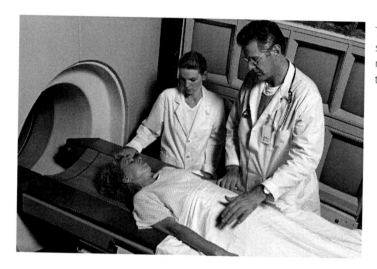

The clinical development of sensitive neuroimaging agents requires carefully designed clinical trials.

What happens before we embark on a drug trial?

Pharmaceutical R&D (Research and Development) can be broken into two parts: drug discovery and drug development. The overarching aim is to produce a new drug that is commercially and medically of value, and preferably one that is easy to make, easy to administer, pure, sterile, and stable. There are many areas of expertise involved, from biochemistry and pharmacology, through to chemistry and engineering. Pharmaceutical companies create teams that integrate these skills. These teams follow a basic process, which can be broken into the following steps:

Target identification

This is the medical indications (condition/illness/disease etc) for which the company hopes to develop a product, and the underlying pharmacology or the mechanism of action of the drug they believe will have the desired medical effect. As an example, a company might target developing a new oral analgesic known as an NSAID (non-steroid anti-inflammatory drug), with reduced incidence of gastric ulceration. Scientists in this case (inside or outside the company) would have determined this meant they needed an inhibitor that was specific for the "prostaglandin cyclo-oxygenase type II" enzyme – involved in the local perception of pain. This inhibitor would need to have only a limited effect on the type I enzyme (which has other functions in the stomach and inhibition of which tends to lead to gastric ulceration). This may have been the way the target of the so-called COX-2 inhibitors were born, ultimately leading to some of the world's most useful, profitable (and ultimately controversial) products.

> Target identification: the identification of medical indications ... for which the company hopes to develop a product, and the underlying pharmacology or the mechanism of action of the drug they believe will have the desired medical effect.

As a second example, a company may decide that medicine needs a way to prevent the degeneration of joints in rheumatoid arthritis. Scientists would have determined that the action of a cytokine called TNF (Tumor Necrosis Factor) Alpha may be critical in the process of joint destruction. They could choose one of several ways to inhibit this action, perhaps by preventing production of the cytokine, or by preventing its action on cellular mechanism, or by speeding up its natural destruction. Different companies will choose different techniques based on their expertise. Several companies decided to attempt the production of 'biologic' drugs – in this case an antibody specific to TNF Alpha to bind to the cytokine and prevent it having its action.

Lead identification

Using whatever tools the company favors (see table 1), scientists will create a series of biological products or smaller synthetic molecules they believe will have the desired properties. This can take a very long time, may never happen, or can be relatively simple. The COX-2 example above could have taken many years. Biologicals however, can be very fast. In our TNF Alpha example, the creation of antibodies specific to the molecule is a well understood process which may take only a few months.

Lead optimization

Once a chemical or biological product is found that seems to demonstrate the desired effect it needs to be refined. A 'series' of similar products is created, each with small variations, and tested against a variety of objectives. This process is a balancing act, trying to find the best in the series for properties such as:

✦ *Receptor specificity* – In the examples above, we are trying to find which 'small molecule' produces the most COX-2 inhibition and the least COX-1 inhibitions, or which 'biological' produces the best removal of TNF Alpha?

✦ *Initial safety in animals* – Which of the series produce the least damage to the physiological systems of test animals?

✦ *Simplicity and scalability of the synthetic route* – is it relatively easy and inexpensive to make the drug in bulk?

TABLE 1

High throughput screening

The process is a mixture of biology, robotics and computational science, designed to rapidly and automatically test the hundreds and thousands of new chemicals, looking for specific pharmacological actions. Essentially it is the process of looking for a needle in a haystack at such a speed that results are obtained in reasonable time frames. The system is fed by the use of combinational chemistry (a set of tools and techniques capable of producing thousands of new chemical structures quickly), and chemical libraries (a set of tools designed to track the creation of such chemicals and record their structure and other properties so they can be reproduced). Once the chemicals are produced they are tested in production line style across a battery of tests designed to show if any of them has an effect on a target molecular mechanism that is predicted to have a medical impact – perhaps an inhibitor of a certain enzyme, or blockade of a certain receptor, etc.

These tools require huge investment of several billion dollars which can only be afforded by large companies. These systems have replaced more traditional methods, although there is little hard evidence as yet that the expected benefits will materialize.

Traditional methods

These are still the mainstay of small companies and biotech companies:

Natural product screening

Where companies look for plants used by local populations for specific medical conditions, and try to isolate the active product.

Rational development

Where scientists use published and private information to make their own assessments of what chemical structures will produce the desired effects – then produce and test those elements to refine their ideas until they find one that works.

✦ *Oral activity* – drugs that can be swallowed are more likely to do well in the market than those that need to be injected.

✦ *Duration of effect* – drugs that need to be taken only once a day are more likely to do well in the market than those taken, say, four times a day.

Once tested the best of the series of similar products is selected and moved into development. The safety pharmacology is assessed in animals in more depth and the way they react to the new drug is explored. In particular we need to know how the body will handle the foreign element (the drug) – specifically how it is absorbed; what concentration it reaches in the blood and elsewhere in the body, and how quickly concentrations are reached; how the drug is broken down and removed and by which organ (liver? kidney?). All this information helps plan how the drug should be used in humans. After these tests, there ensues a set of toxicology studies designed to weed out drugs that may cause significant harm to humans. We can do this by watching the drug's longer-term effects on animals.

To start our clinical trials we need to know that the product is safe, sterile, pure, as well as how long it will be stable on the shelf – as some of our studies can be quite long – and whether it needs to be kept in special containers – for example to keep out light or moisture. The company's pharmaceutical research group produces all of this information, in parallel with the work done on animal studies, so the best possible chemical product and formulation (all the other material added to the active ingredient to create a pill or injection) is available for the clinical trials to start.

> To start our clinical trials we need to know that this product is safe, sterile, pure, as well as how long it will be stable on the shelf…

Conducting clinical trials

The entire aim of our present clinical trials system is to provide data that is accurate and honest. The data should quantify the safety and efficacy (effectiveness) of the drug so medical practitioners can use it appropriately.

The beginning of this chapter identified two major concepts that underpin trial design and structure. First, that trials are scientific experiments, and second that measuring medical outcomes is complex. These concepts require further explanation:

Clinical trials are experiments

Any experiment has to ask a question. Early in a drug's development the questions being asked are typically basic. They become more complex and detailed as information accumulates. The development of the questions is managed by creating an overall plan for the development of the drug from its first use in humans right through to an application for a license to market the product (granted by each country's regulatory agency for medicines) and beyond. This 'development plan' lays out the anticipated program of trials, each taking the knowledge about the drug to a new level. Once the medicine is on the market, the development of

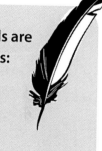

Clinical trials are experiments: Any experiment has to ask a question.

further knowledge continues, but is much less controlled, because although the company selling the product will continue to run a defined program, trials will also be run by many other organizations for their own purposes.

Initial questions to be addressed by clinical trials may include:

+ Is the drug safe? Trials assess the risks associated with taking the drug and the best way to use it.
+ Is the drug effective? Trials assess the benefits and overall value of the drug.

Once these basic questions are addressed, then more complex questions can be approached, such as:

+ What dose provides the optimum balance of risk (safety) and benefit (efficacy)?
+ How often should the drug be given?
+ Is the use of this drug cost effective?
+ What place should the drug have in the present treatment algorithms (should the drug be the first that a physician prescribes, or only used when others fail)?
+ What types or sub groups of patients will get the most benefit?
+ How does the drug compare to other medications for a specific indication (the defined illness or condition)?
+ What should the drug cost?

Common elements in trials

Whatever the questions asked, all trials have to ensure the safety of the patient and the integrity of the data. To achieve these goals, commercial and (recently) non-commercial trials have to conform to certain standards. These standards are called 'Good Clinical Practice' or GCP, the various versions of which were 'harmonized' (agreed) between regulatory agencies from the USA, Japan and Europe, and pharmaceutical companies some years ago. They have since passed into various forms of legislation around the world.

> ... [A]ll trials have to ensure the safety of the patient and the integrity of the data. To achieve this commercial and (recently) non-commercial trials have to conform to certain standards, codified as 'Good Clinical Practice' or GCP.

Generally, all trials also conform to the World Medical Association's Declaration of Helsinki – a statement issued in 1964 of the requirements of ethical treatment of patients first introduced after the Second World War as a response to the unethical experimentation by the Nazis on various types of people. The declaration has been updated many times, the most recent of which introduced a vast array of detail previously not included, which has led to significant controversy and some trials stating they conform only to earlier versions. Whichever version is used however, GCP and the Helsinki declaration protect patients by ensuring all clinical trials:

+ Have ethics committee approval[1].
+ Ensure patients provide informed consent to participate in the trial.
+ Inform participants how their data will be used.
+ Allow patients to drop out at any time, for no reason.
+ Do not prejudice the quality of treatment the patient will get.
+ Allow each patient the potential to benefit personally from the new treatment under investigation.

---

1 [Ed] An ethics committee should consist of a reasonable number of members with the collective qualifications to review and evaluate the science, medical and ethical aspects of the proposed trial. Ethics committees tend to be representative of the communities they serve. They include members of both gender, at least one lay person from the community with no affiliations with the institution, member(s) with knowledge of the areas of research, and those with medical or psychological, and legal training.

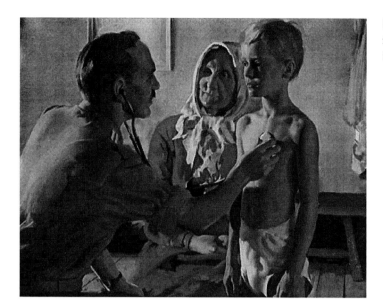

International guidelines exist to safeguard and protect participants involved in clinical trials.

The codification of GCP is voluminous, so cannot be reviewed in detail here. However, the general principles are straightforward: that the patient should at all times remain safe, and that the data collected are complete and accurate. All the rules flow from these two principles:

Patient safety

Standardized processes are used when evaluating clinical trial safety events. Common criteria are agreed on that may be potentially 'serious'. This means that all trials run fairly standard assessments of Serious Adverse Events (SAEs). The investigators at the hospitals conducting the clinical trials have an obligation to report such adverse events to the sponsoring company within 24 hours. The company must have a system for reporting serious adverse events deemed related to the drug within 7 to 15 days, and for reporting all events at regular periods during the development of the drug.

Data integrity

The accuracy and completeness of data is managed in a number of ways: by ensuring that the patients actually exist, and that patient data has been accurately recorded by checking a percentage of key data against their hospital or primary care notes and other medical records (Source Data Verification). The Data Managers run a series of sense checks and data cleaning programs over the database to raise queries about the data, which are then returned to the investigators and resolved and re-recorded.

Classifying clinical trials

All clinical trials are unique, designed to answer a specific question. The document that describes how the trial will be conducted is called a protocol. Many components of these documents are the same from trial to trial, especially for the same intervention and in the same patient populations. However, elements of the protocol that define the unique parts of the trial should be written from scratch, as too much reliance on templates and boilerplate text can lead to a poor study design that may fail to address the question it was intended to answer.

Classifying trials is often based on those elements they have in common. The most common classifications are:

1. Phase
2. Objective
3. Endpoint

> **All clinical trials are unique, designed to answer a specific question. The document that describes how the trial will be conducted is called a protocol.**

Classified by Phase

While this is the oldest and mostly commonly used classification, it is not particularly useful as it does not convey much information about the trial.

Phase I – human volunteers. The trials are undertaken in volunteers – usually young healthy males. Initial doses are tiny, building up slowly to larger single doses and then to multiple doses to the same person, over the space of several days or weeks. The aim is to determine whether the product is tolerated by humans in the doses expected to be used and to measure basic medical parameters to monitor any acute (immediate) side effects. We then measure the pharmacokinetics of the drug, which tell us how the body's systems handle the drug – how well it is absorbed, what blood levels are achieved, what other parts of the body does it reach, where in the body it is broken down or metabolized, how is it excreted, etc.

Phase II – early patient trials. Once the drug is shown to be safe in healthy volunteers, it is given to patients to see if it actually works. Trials at this stage are still small, so definitive statistical evidence of a clinical effect may not be possible. At this point, exposure needs to be limited as knowledge on the safety of the product is low. The aim is to gradually increase the number of patients treated and duration of exposure (a day, a week, a month of therapy for example), checking for safety and looking for an effect on the condition to ensure the product is still worth developing. The single most important question to be answered in this phase is that of dose – what is the best dose to study in the forthcoming large scale exposure studies and then, hopefully, place on the market.

Phase III – large scale exposure of patients. Once a few hundred patients have taken the drug it becomes sensible to increase the degree of exposure significantly. To demonstrate subtle differences between therapies you need more patients, hence it takes large studies to really compare the product against its future competitors. This makes Phase III the most important from both a marketing and a safety perspective. These are the last trials prior to an application for a license to market the drug, and will continue until the product is approved or rejected.

Phase IV – trials after a license has been granted. This covers any trial once a marketing authorization has been granted. They are carried out for a huge number of reasons and come in many different shapes and sizes. They can be very large safety studies looking for rare side effects, or small studies aimed at looking at very specific actions of the drug.

Classified by Objective

Every trial has a brief description of its objectives. These objectives put it into a much larger set of more informative categories. The categories most commonly used (although not an exhaustive list) are described in the table, mapped against their usual place in the phasing categories. These categories have descriptive titles, so they tell us much more about a trial and are therefore better when trying to communicate the purpose of a trial to interested parties.

Below are common categories and descriptions:

- ✦ First in Man – the first time a human is exposed
- ✦ Pharmacokinetic – usually absolute measurements regarding the behavior of the drug in the body
- ✦ Proof of concept – setting up a simple test for the effect being sought. For example giving a volunteer a pain stimulus and then seeing if this is reduced by a drug you hope is an analgesic
- ✦ Mechanism of action – looking for the pharmacological effect of a product - eg. receptor blockade
- ✦ Dose ranging – exploring the doses required for maximum effect with minimum side effects
- ✦ Large scale exposure – the large trials in actual patient populations looking at safety and efficacy in detail
- ✦ Expanded access – studies designed to increase the exposure of patients to a product as it comes up to licensing
- ✦ Peri-launch – trials around the launch of the drug to maximize its commercial impact when launched
- ✦ Regulatory committment – a trial required by the licensing authority in order to approve the license
- ✦ Market support – trials to meet the needs of the prescribing physicians who are experts in their field

Research Groups are likely to place ads in the local newspapers seeking volunteers for their study.

The following table summarizes the classification of clinical trials by their broad objectives as described above.

Table 2: Classification of clinical trials by objective.

Phase	Broad Objectives
Phase I	FIM (first in man)
	PK (pharmacokinetic)
Phase I or II	Proof of concept
	Mechanism of Action
Phase II	Dose Ranging
Phase III	Large scale exposure
Phase IIIb (late phase III)	Expanded access
Phase IIIb moving to IV	Peri-launch
Phase IV	Regulatory commitment
	Market support data

Classified by Endpoint

An endpoint is an outcome measured in the trial and is either pharmacokinetic or pharmacodynamic.

Pharmacokinetic (PK) endpoints are usually absolute measurements regarding the behavior of the drug in the body – for example, the *time* taken to reach peak concentration in the blood, the final concentration it reaches in a key area of the body (perhaps the synovial fluid in the joint or the cerebro-spinal fluid surrounding the brain and spinal cord), the amount of the drug absorbed by the gut, the amount excreted by the kidneys, etc.

Pharmacodynamic endpoints reflect the action of the drug. These can be closely or distantly related to the signs and symptoms the patients suffers. For example, when studying an angiotensin inhibitor for hypertension, you can:

✦ measure the activity of angiotensin in the blood before and after dosing – often called a pharmacological endpoint
✦ measure the blood pressure after multiple doses – a surrogate endpoint
✦ measure the final impact of the condition, such as the number of strokes and heart attacks suffered – an outcome endpoint.

Each type of endpoint has advantages and disadvantages. Pharmacological endpoints tend to be fast and simple but they are unable to demonstrate if the desired medical effect is achieved. More medical information comes from surrogate endpoints, because these measurements must be known to relate to the severity of the medical condition, but will usually require longer exposure. Outcome measures continue this trend, representing the ultimate in medical relevance, providing unarguable proof of effect, but will take a considerable length of time to demonstrate.

Elements of experimental design and structure

Trials often have long descriptive titles which define the elements of how they have been designed, providing an insight into the purpose and potential ways to interpret the results. There are two key elements of design usually covered: how you control the study, and how you structure the groups of patients compared.

Control

A study usually compares the effect of a therapy on two or more groups of patients. Each group has to be treated as much as possible identically except for the different therapy. Therefore each group follows the same schedule, takes medications that look the same, gets the same tests that are done in the same way, sometimes even by the same people, using the same criteria for assessment. The main question here is what should we compare the new medicine against? Commonly used approaches are to compare against:

+ nothing
+ an alternative specified therapy
+ a basket of therapies that represent the 'best practice' for each individual patient.

To remove bias in recording results, neither the patient nor physician should know what therapy the patient is taking, so the control patient is given dummy (placebo) medication. If the drug is being compared to no therapy, then this is simple – the placebo is the same tablet as that being tested, minus the active ingredient. However, if the new drug is being compared to an existing, active therapy, then, to ensure no one knows which is being taken, patients in each group must take both types of medicine. To illustrate this, in one group, therapy A will be active, and therapy B will be the dummy, and in the other group the reverse, A is dummy, B is active. This ensures both the patient and physician are blind to the therapy for an individual patient – the so called double dummy, double blind design. In some cases it is not possible or safe to create a placebo / dummy, and in that case the physician will usually know what therapy the patient is on, but not the patient. This is called single blind. It may also be impossible to create any form of blinding, so the patient also knows what therapy they are on. These are termed 'open' design studies.

When assessing the results of a trial it is important to know the methods of control and comparison. Open studies have more potential for bias, and so their data is less reliable. They offer less certainty of the outcome, so if treatment differences are small, open design studies may not be as believable. The more control you introduce, the more you can reduce the opportunity for (so-called *confounding*) differences between the treatment groups you are assessing. This reduces the variability in the study data, making it more likely to show the drug effect you are looking for. The most credible results tend to come from double blind, randomized, placebo controlled or double dummy studies.

Group structures.

Study groups have to be as similar as possible before therapy starts. This is achieved by allocating patients to therapy groups randomly. However, some variations are possible, such as stratification, matched groups and cross-over designs.

Stratification is used when patients entering the study come from two or more distinct groups. For example, in a hypertension study some patients may be on nitrate therapy, some not. Stratification ensures the two study groups have the same number taking nitrates, allowing the nitrate effects to cancel out.

Matched groups are used when there are a number of other variables that might affect the outcome of the study. In this case, an individual in one group is matched for those variables as much as possible with an individual in the other group, increasing the similarity of the groups when they start. For example if age and sex might affect the response to a therapy, then patients are matched for these two variables in each group.

Cross over designs take this one step further. Patients in each group take first one therapy, and are evaluated. They then take the other therapy. In this way, the two groups are made up of the same patients – in essence they are perfectly matched.

Measuring medical parameters

Direct measurements

All of the methods mentioned above need specialized statistical treatment. Clinical scientists look for medical parameters they can measure that help answer the clinical questions being investigated. Trials tend to use the standard medical assessments of the severity and characteristics of a condition. These are based on:

✦ symptoms (what the patient tells us)

✦ signs (what the medical practitioner observes).

✦ Investigations (blood tests, X-rays, lung function tests, ECGs, etc.)

As an example, in a rheumatoid (painful joints) study we can ask the patient the general question, "do you feel better?" Or we may ask the physician, "do you think the patient is better?" We record the answer as a number using a variety of techniques. A common example is the Visual Analog Scale. The patient or physician is asked to mark on a 10cm line the point which they think best represents the answer to the question. They may use a scale between the two extremes of "never been so bad" at one end (the 'zero' end) and "never been so good" at 10cm end. We then measure how far along the line the answer is recorded. Many variations on these scoring systems exist – perhaps just allocating a score of 1 to 5, or answering a set of questions and adding up scores for different answers. Many of these measures are actually very reproducible, but the number generated has no intrinsic meaning – it is a subjective score. To supplement these measurements we therefore ask other objective questions. For example, in our rheumatoid example a 'joint count' may be used, where the patient indicates which of his or her joints are painful (just hurt all the time), tender (hurt when pressed), swollen or hot and inflamed (red). This produces a lot of numbers, each of which has intrinsic meaning about the condition. The disadvantage to this method is that the numbers don't tell you how the patient is actually feeling. The true power of the measures comes when they are combined.

We can also measure many other parameters. For rheumatoid these include levels of natural elements in the blood such as CRP (C-reactive protein) and the size and shape of joints as seen by X-ray or MRI (Magnetic Resonance Imaging). Each indication will have as many of these assessments as can be made.

Combining measurements

A key medical question for any patient is their prognosis. This involves predicting how their condition will progress and what impact the treatments will have. Often, to get the best prediction of disease outcome, we aggregate several measures to create categories of severity of disease, which have been shown to have different prognoses. We can use these categories in clinical trials, measuring the numbers of patients moved between categories by a therapy. If a drug tends to move patients to a less severe category then we assume the drug improves the overall prognosis of those patients that move, telling us something meaningful about the future of the patient, as well as the present state of their condition and the benefits of the drug.

Not all aggregate categories are used for prognosis. Physicians also use measures to create categories of patients who will respond to different therapies (e.g. who might get severe side effects or respond well using different therapeutic approaches). Clinical trials are a key tool used to produce these categories, and so may assess different categorization techniques as part of their outcome measures. If a trial uses a new technique, the regulatory authorities require such measures to be 'validated'. Validation means you have to have evidence – your own or that of others – that shows such measures can correlate to disease severity or to absolute outcomes we can all regard as valuable – such as more years of pain-free life.

Weaknesses in trials

Despite our best efforts, there are some inherent weaknesses in clinical trials that need to be understood to interpret their results correctly. Some of these weaknesses include the following.

1. Trials are highly controlled environments and run on samples of the population. How we extrapolate their data to cover the broader population of patients is determined by the regulatory agencies and groups who control whether a medicine is placed on a formulary. The actual patients who will be using the product are more varied, and many may not respond as expected. Post license studies (e.g., phase IV) address this issue to a degree, as the objectives for trials are broader and not focused purely on achieving a license.

2. Pharmacovigilance (the long term monitoring of safety of drugs in use in the population) is also important, as it allows us to spot if unpredicted side effects are occuring in the much larger and broader population now taking the medication.

3. Informed consent can be fraught with ethical issues, because it is subjective. 'Informed' is taken to imply understanding. Many patients do not understand complex medical issues, yet of course they are entitled to take part in trials if they desire. In an attempt to improve consent, detailed descriptions of the experience with the drug and recorded side effects are produced in consent forms – although there is no guarantee this actually increases the patients' understanding.

4. Investigators, nurses, pharmaceutical staff and all number of other staff are paid for the time they spend with patients in trials, so you cannot escape the possibility of bias in recommending patients to be included, and in rare cases that patients may be recruited in a fraudulent way.

5. Studies are audited by the regulatory agencies and a large number of independent Quality Assurance contractors or staff within pharmaceutical companies to provide an independent review of the quality and integrity of the data collected. Those infringing the rules can be severely punished. However, fraud still exists to a limited degree.

6. Lastly, a highly regulated environment is necessary to ensure minimum levels of operational quality. However, this environment also tends to reduce innovation and freedom of thinking – effectively pushing standards to an agreed but minimum level. Following a quality process because we are told to do so can be less effective than controlling quality by creating a process we have designed for the specific situation.

Many pharmaceutical companies have introduced Quality Management Systems – their own commercially driven approach to quality – to supplement external systems.

In summary

Clinical trials are carried out once a product has been through extensive pre-clinical investigation. This is part of the discovery process in most pharmaceutical companies. The discovery process includes target disease identification, definition of molecular classes of drugs that might be used in therapy, and the search for a chemical with those properties. After a suitable candidate is found, it is assessed for basic safety, and for the desired effect in animals. The drug candidate is then tested in humans.

Clinical trials are complex experiments run in humans to determine the effect of an intervention on the medical status of a group of individuals. Clinical trial plans include the overall investigation of the product prior to registration, and sometimes after they are marketed. They start by asking and answering simple questions. They progress to more complex assessments as we learn more about the drug, how it can be used, what patients benefit from it, and how it compares with other products that might be used for the same condition.

Initially, trials start with tiny doses given to healthy volunteers (Phase I). They progress to early assessments in patients to evaluate that the mechanism of action is as expected, and that there are at least indications that the desired effect may be present (Phase II). Dose is determined at this point, and the product is then passed into large scale Phase III trials to assess the drug's benefits and risks and to compare it to other treatments on the market. Once completed, all the data are gathered into a dossier for application for a drug license. If approved by the regulatory authorities the product is launched. Any Phase IV trial would start at this point, when the product is approved, and run until the product is eventually replaced by a better therapy, or otherwise withdrawn from the market.

Trial design is focused around the proper control of variability in the study through randomization and blinding, structure of the groups to be compared, and the obvious benefits and risks expected from their use.

Regulation of trials is tight. Medical expertise and training ensures patients are always treated in their own best interests, and external organizations – mostly regulatory agencies from various major markets, such as the FDA in the U.S. – check that the clinical trial process is running according to various rules and regulations, mostly captured within GCP.

Chapter 2

FDA and clinical drug trials: a short history

Suzanne White Junod, Ph.D.[1]

Food and Drug Administration, USA

> "The function of the controlled clinical trial is not the "discovery" of a new drug or therapy. Discoveries are made in the animal laboratory, by chance observation, or at the bedside by an acute clinician. The function of the formal controlled clinical trial is to separate the relative handful of discoveries which prove to be true advances in therapy from a legion of false leads and unverifiable clinical impressions, and to delineate in a scientific way the extent of and the limitations which attend the effectiveness of drugs."
>
> — *William Thomas Beaver*[2]

Overview

The U.S. Food and Drug Administration (FDA) has evolved as one of the world's foremost institutional authorities for conducting and evaluating controlled clinical drug trials.

Ancient civilizations relied on medical observation to identify herbs, drugs and therapies that worked, and those that did not. Beginning in the early twentieth century, therapeutic reformers in the United States and in other places began to develop the concept of the "well-controlled" therapeutic drug trial. This concept included, for example, laboratory analysis followed by clinical study. As medical historians have pointed out, however, these early reformers' therapeutic vision often far exceeded their clinical and experimental grasp.[3] In 1938, a newly enacted U.S. Food, Drug, and Cosmetic Act subjected new drugs to pre-market safety evaluation for the first time. This required FDA regulators to review both pre-clinical and clinical test results for new drugs. Although the law did not specify the kinds of tests that were required for approval, the new authority allowed drug officials to block the marketing of a new drug formally or delay it by requiring additional data. The Act also gave regulators limited powers of negotiation over scientific study and approval requirements with the pharmaceutical industry and the medical profession. A worldwide drug disaster in 1961 resulted in the enactment of the 1962 Drug Amendments, which explicitly stated that the FDA would rely on scientific testing and that new drug approvals would be based not only on proof of safety, but also on 'substantial evidence' of a drug's efficacy [i.e., the impact of a drug in a clinical trial setting]. Increasingly, responsibility for testing standards, previously established as voluntary by the American Medical Association's (AMA) Council on Drugs, the U.S. Pharmacopeia (USP) and the National Formulary, were taken up by the FDA. Since 1962, the FDA has overseen substantial refinements to the broad legal requirement that post-1962 new drugs be approved on the basis of 'adequate and well-controlled' studies.[4]

> The U.S. Food and Drug Administration (FDA) has evolved as one of the world's foremost institutional authorities for conducting and evaluating controlled clinical drug trials.

Medical observation as precursor to clinical trials

Clinical trials are prospective, organized, systematic exposures of patients to an intervention of some kind (drug, surgical procedure, dietary change). The earliest recorded therapeutic investigations, however, lacked the rigor of a modern clinical trial. Based largely on observations and tested through time by trial and error, ancient medicine such as that practiced by the Egyptians, Babylonians, and Hebrews was closely allied with religion. Nonetheless, some of these early medical investigations did yield some important successes in fields such as minor surgery and orthopedics. The Hebrews, in particular, excelled in public hygiene, but even their public health strictures, so effective in preventing epidemic disease, were observational and experiential rather than experimental.[5]

> Clinical trials are prospective, organized, systematic exposures of patients to an intervention of some kind (drug, surgical procedure, dietary change).

The Babylonians reportedly exhibited their sick in a public place so that onlookers could freely offer their therapeutic advice based on previous and personal experience.[6] The first mention of a paid experimental subject came from diarist Samuel Pepys who documented an experiment involving a paid subject in a diary entry for November 21, 1667. He noted that the local college had hired a "poor and debauched man" to have some sheep blood "let into his body." Although there had been plenty of consternation beforehand, the man apparently suffered no ill effects.

One of the most memorable successes from an early but earnest clinical trial was actually more of an anomaly rather than a harbinger of great progress in medical experimentation. British naval surgeon James Lind (1716-1794), who had learned of the death of three quarters of a ships' crew during a long voyage around the world, planned a comparative trial of several popularly suggested "cures" for the scurvy on his next voyage. Twelve men with similar cases of scurvy ate a common diet and slept together. Six pairs, however, were given different "treatments" for their malady. Two were given a quart of cider daily; two an "elixir;" two seawater; two a remedy suggested by the ship's surgeon (horseradish, mustard and garlic);

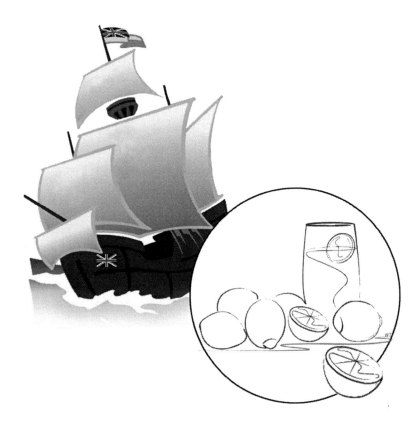

British naval surgeon James Lind (1716-1794) planned a comparative trial of several popularly suggested "cures" for scurvy on a voyage around the world. His experiment with "oranges and lemons" produced a positive result that caused the British Navy to supply citrus to its ships.

two vinegar; and the final two were given "oranges and lemons" daily. One man who received the oranges and lemons recovered within six days, while the other recovered sufficiently that he "was appointed nurse to the rest of the sick." At first Lind questioned his own experimental results, but by the time he published them (1753 and 1757) they were recognized as important. Nonetheless, the British Navy did not supply citrus to its ships until 1795.[7]

Although simple observation may provide a starting point for medical study, experience has shown that it is rarely efficient at advancing medical knowledge. As one early proponent of planned experimentation in the form of clinical trials remarked, "when we are reduced to [mere] observation, science crawls."[8] A modern drug regulator is more explicit, acknowledging that modern retrospective [studies], epidemiologic analyses, and astute observations are all instructive. However, clinical trials are not the only way to find things out. "But, the clinical trial is unique in being under the investigator's control, subject not to data availability or chance but to his ability to ask good questions and design means of answering them."[9]

Evolution of clinical trial concept in America

According to medical historian Harry Marks, the modern controlled clinical trial is largely an American invention as statistically-based clinical trials became a critically important part of evidence-based medicine in the U.S. following WWII.[10] Certainly clinical trials in this country have evolved in pursuit of a larger therapeutic goal -- to see that physicians use the best possible therapies available. It is interesting to note that in the late 19th century, U.S. animal rights activists protested against the use of human beings as subjects in medical experiments. In their quest to protect animals, they viewed both animals and human beings as equally vulnerable, and feared that the replacement of the family physician by a "scientist at the bedside" would inspire non-therapeutic experimentation. It was the antivivisectionist and playwright George Bernard Shaw, in fact, who first used the term "human guinea pig."[11]

> In 1880, patent medicines… constituted 28% of marketed drugs. By 1900, however, they represented 72% of drug sales and products with inert ingredients were promoted vigorously.

Nonetheless, as early as the late nineteenth and early twentieth century, interest in clinical objectivity grew, spurred on not only by astounding successes in laboratory science and clinical medicine abroad (e.g. discovery of microbes, pasteurization of milk, development of anthrax and rabies vaccines) but because of the sorry state of therapeutics at the time in America. In 1880, patent medicines – a misnomer because nothing but the label and the bottle were actually patented or trademarked – constituted 28% of marketed drugs. By 1900, however, they represented 72% of drug sales and products with inert ingredients were promoted as vigorously, if not more so, than drugs with active ingredients. It was popular to blame both the gullible physician and the ignorant laymen for being equally taken in by the advertising excesses of the era.[12]

The American Medical Association (AMA) began to push for federal evaluation of new medical products hoping to make a dent in the patent medicine industry, but it was unsuccessful. In 1905, the AMA formed its own Council on Pharmacy and Chemistry, which levied a fee on manufacturers to evaluate their drugs for quality (ingredient testing) and safety. Drugs accepted by the Council could carry the AMA's Seal of Acceptance and only products with the seal had access to the advertising pages of the *Journal of the American Medical Association* (JAMA). The AMA's Chemical Laboratory tested commercial statements about the composition and purity of drugs in their labs, while the Council on Pharmacy and Chemistry followed up with safety and rudimentary efficacy evaluations designed to eliminate exaggerated or misleading therapeutic claims.[13] Although the Council eagerly sought evidence that drugs had an effect on the cause or course of a disease, the Seal was awarded to drugs that merely provided symptomatic relief. The Council would have liked to rely on clinical studies to supplement laboratory studies submitted by drug manufacturers, but they lacked the necessary funding to support such studies and the AMA did not authorize the Council to require them. Instead of relying on the anecdotal information provided by private practitioners, however, the Council relied heavily on the opinions and recommendations of Council members who were well-respected medical specialists and scientists, a progressive practice for the era. Once their evaluations became a regular feature in the Journal of the American Medical Association (JAMA) the Council began to make inroads against the commercialism that physicians had felt were 'debauching' medical journals and 'tainting' medical textbooks. The AMA's drug certification program remained in place until 1955.

Clinical trials and the 1906 Pure Food and Drugs Act

While the AMA Council on Pharmacy and Chemistry held out the carrot of certification to ethical drug products that met their standards, the first federal food and drug statute, the 1906 Pure Food and Drugs Act, wielded little in the way of a stick. The AMA had been unsuccessful in getting any kind of drug review in the new law and the statute merely provided a legal definition for the terms 'adulterated' and 'misbranded' as they related to both food and drug products and prescribed legal penalties for each offense. The law did empower the Bureau of Chemistry (forerunner of the U.S. Food and Drug Administration) to seize adulterated and misbranded products that moved in interstate commerce, but it simply adopted the drug standards as published in the U.S. Pharmacopeia and the National Formulary. The law also prohibited "false and misleading" statements on product labels. In the case of drugs, the law listed eleven so-called "dangerous ingredients" including opium (and its derivatives) and alcohol, which, if they were present in the product, had to be listed on the drug label. This listing requirement alone inspired many manufacturers to abandon use of many dangerous ingredients following passage of the 1906 Act. But efforts to prohibit false therapeutic claims on drug labels were defeated both by the Supreme Court and in the U.S. Congress.

During the 1920's, 30's and 40's medical researchers began to conduct "cooperative investigations" designed to overcome errors attributed to individual observers working in relative isolation and replace them with standardized evaluations of therapeutic research in hundreds of patients.[14] Therapeutic experimentation, however, did not begin to gain a true foothold in modern medicine until the U.S. legal system stopped equating experimentation with medical malpractice. As late as 1934, state courts seemed to uphold traditional views that the doctor was bound to act within accepted methods of clinical practice and that patients had not consented for their physician to deviate from these methods.[15] In a landmark state Supreme Court decision in 1935, however, the state of Michigan seemed to recognize and authorize controlled clinical investigations as a part of medical practice without subjecting the researcher to strict liability (without fault) for any injury so long as the patient consented to the experiment and it did not "vary too radically" from accepted methods of procedure.[16] In particular, the Michigan Supreme Court accepted that experimentation was necessary not just to treat the individual, but also to help medicine progress. "We recognize," noted the Court, "the fact that if the general practice of medicine and surgery is to progress, there must be a certain amount of experimentation carried on."

> During the 1920's, 30's and 40's medical researchers began to conduct "cooperative investigations" designed to overcome errors attributed to individual observers working in relative isolation…

By 1937, it had become clear to regulators and to an increasing number of outside organizations, including the AMA, that the original 1906 'Wiley' Act had become outdated. Breakthrough drugs such as the first sulfa drug, sulfanilamide, new drugs including amphetamines and biologics such as insulin were coming onto the market and beginning to transform medicine entirely. Clinical trials and human experimentation were becoming increasingly more important in medical research. Moreover, turn-of-the-century patent medicines with inert ingredients and quirky but quaint labels were becoming a true public health danger when patients relied on them rather than seeking out effective new therapies. The case of Banbar, in particular, convinced regulators early in the 1930's that the 1906 law's recognition of the rights of proprietors was becoming an increasing impediment to efforts to insure drug safety.

Soon after the 1906 Act had been enacted, a dispute arose over the meaning and enforcement of the drug labeling provisions of the law. The Supreme Court ruled in *U.S. v. Johnson* in 1911, that the new law did not prohibit false therapeutic claims – the product involved was labeled Dr. Johnson's Cure for Cancer – it just prohibited "false and misleading" label claims regarding the ingredients or identity of the drug. In 1912, Congress quickly enacted the Sherley Amendment, a compromise that merely prohibited false therapeutic claims "intended to defraud" the consumer. Proving that a proprietor knew that a drug was worthless in order to demonstrate fraud under the statute, however, could be a daunting task. To cite a single example: an old patent medicine maker created a 'cure' for diabetes which he marketed as Banbar. Its active ingredients included milk sugar and equisetum (horsetail). The product was particularly dangerous since diabetics were rejecting insulin injections in favor of Banbar (the hormone insulin had been isolated in 1922 and was a lifesaving therapy for diabetics). FDA seized the Banbar product in the mid-1930s, charging the proprietor with fraud under the Sherley Amendment. In his defense, the proprietor submitted testimonial letters written to him thanking him for the product. His lawyer argued that it was obvious, since these

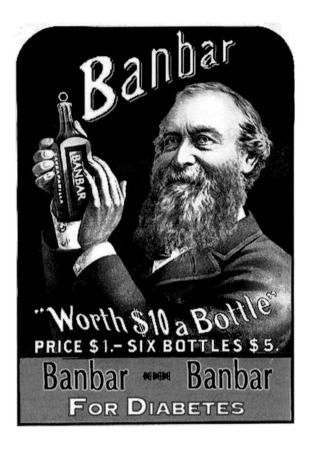

An old patent medicine maker created a 'cure' for diabetes which he marketed as Banbar.

sincere people took the trouble to write him and thank him, that he had no idea that the product might not be effective, much less dangerous. Government officials selected a representative group of testimonial letters and matched them side-by-side with death certificates from the same individuals indicating that they had died from diabetes. Although the public health threat was obvious, the court ruled that the proprietor had not intended to defraud his customers and the product remained on the market until Congress enacted a new food and drug statute without this so-called 'fraud joker' in 1938. Banbar, in particular, gave drug regulators their first direct experience interpreting drug data obtained not from direct clinical trials, but from both uncontrolled trials and 'historical' data, one of three types of clinical trial data eventually recognized as acceptable under law in 1970.[17]

Most consumers were unaware of Banbar, but in 1937, a broader drug disaster did capture public attention and first drew the federal government into playing a limited, but soon growing role in the evaluation of new drugs, including the conduct of clinical trials for new drugs. In 1937 a drug company developed a liquid preparation of the first 'wonder drug' sulfanilamide, used to fight streptococcal infections (i.e. strep throat). The product was not tested in animals or humans prior to marketing. The solvent used to suspend the active drug, diethylene glycol, was a poison (chemically related to anti-freeze). It required the entire field force of the FDA to retrieve all available bottles of Elixir Sulfanilamide when the company's own recall efforts proved inadequate to the task. FDA, however, was only empowered to act against the deadly product because it was misbranded -- it contained no alcohol whereas the term 'elixir' implied that it did contain alcohol. FDA officials soon discovered that adequate records had not been kept by either physicians or pharmacists documenting prescriptions written and filled for the poisonous product.

Liquid preparation of the first 'wonder drug' sulfanilamide, contained diethylene glycol – a poison (chemically related to anti-freeze). It was marketed to fight streptococcal infections (i.e. strep throat).

Clinical trials and the 1938 Food, Drug, and Cosmetic Act

Congress reacted to the Sulfanilamide tragedy, which killed over 100 people, by enacting a new federal food and drug statute, the 1938 Food, Drug, and Cosmetic Act. A new provision in the act -- requiring drug sponsors to submit safety data to FDA officials for evaluation prior to marketing -- appeared with relatively little discussion following on the heels of the Elixir Sulfanilamide disaster. "Instead of going to market based on their own assessment of the drug, sponsors had to notify the FDA of their intent to market the drug by submitting an NDA (New Drug Application)," explains Dr. Robert Temple, currently head of FDA's Office of Medical Policy. Although the new law did not specify any particular testing method(s), the law did require that drugs be studied by "adequate tests by all methods reasonably applicable to show whether or not the drug is safe." Sponsors were required to demonstrate to FDA that they had carried out all reasonably applicable studies to demonstrate safety and that the drug was "safe for use under the conditions prescribed, recommended or suggested in the proposed labeling thereof."[18] In the future, FDA could use these new tools not only to ban products like Banbar, but to try and prevent drug disasters rather than merely react to them.

> FDA's statutory authority over products increased as a result of egregious public health disasters, but the scientific methodology to evaluate safety and efficacy did not accelerate in tandem.

Under the law, there was no true requirement for FDA 'approval' or 'clearance' of a new drug. Rather, it was presumed that most drugs would be marketed and therefore the default position was 'approval.'[19] Under the 1938 Act, the government had sixty days (which could be extended to 180 days) to complete its safety evaluation. Form 356, the New Drug Application (NDA), required information about all clinical investigations, a full list of the drug's components and composition, methods of manufacture including facilities and controls, and copies of both the packaging and labeling of the new drug. If a company had not received a regulatory response at the end of 60 days it could proceed with marketing its new drug.

Regulators adopted many of the standards and rules of evidence first advocated by turn-of-the-century therapeutic reformers.[20]

Laboratory analysis akin to that originally conducted by the AMA's Chemical Laboratory initially screened most new drugs, companies were required to conduct safety studies, and an increasing number of drugs would soon be studied in the kind of clinical (cooperative) drug trials that the AMA's Council on Pharmacy and Chemistry had advocated, but not conducted, earlier in the century.[21] Animal studies were not required under the 1938 Act to precede human drug trials, but such studies, including animal autopsies, could be requested by regulators as part of the agency's drug safety review. FDA also began to employ the practice, similar to that of the Council, of consulting expert academic specialists, often before making a final decision on drug approvals.[22]

FDA's statutory authority over products increased as a result of egregious public health disasters, but the scientific methodology to evaluate safety and efficacy did not accelerate in tandem. Regulatory work under the new drug safety provisions of the Act was fairly limited, although the new law did sanction factory inspections for the first time and officials were able to eliminate many worthless products submitted for approval to treat serious diseases (i.e. cancer and diabetes) by holding them to be "unsafe" under the statute. Regulators could deny an application if the sponsor's drug application did not include "adequate tests by all methods reasonably applicable to show whether or not such drug is safe for use under the conditions prescribed, recommended or suggested in the proposed labeling thereof."[23] Occasionally, in interpreting this provision, agency officials recommended labeling changes, including warnings, to sponsors and to the U.S.P., but FDA itself lacked authority under the 1938 Act to determine the text and layout of drug labels.[24] Larger efforts to improve drug testing, prescribing patterns, and patient use and compliance, however, were left to the practice of medicine and medicine's scientific and professional authorities.

Although FDA had authority under the 1938 Act to establish rules governing the use of investigational drugs, FDA did not employ this authority to regulate clinical trials and clinical trial methodology until 1961.[25] Even though physicians at elite university clinics and

> **Although FDA had authority under the 1938 Act to establish rules governing the use of investigational drugs, FDA did not employ this authority to regulate clinical trials and clinical trial methodology until 1961.**

members from the AMA Council on Pharmacy and Chemistry all agreed on the importance of standardized drug testing through clinical trials, FDA did not have the authority to require them under the 1938 statute.[26] FDA scientists, however, did begin to exert some influence on the conduct of clinical trials and move in the direction of standardization on the eve of WWII, when they published an article in JAMA on experimental design, proper clinical trial methods, and methods of data analysis.[27] Their article, however, was published as a Report under the auspices of the AMA's Council on Pharmacy and Chemistry and was accompanied by a disclaimer to the effect that the "outline" presented in the report was "offered as an objective, a pattern, and not a regulation." During WWII, the agency actively promoted drug-testing standards in the face of increased wartime expenditures for drug trials designed to answer important questions about the safety and use of many new drugs for the war effort.[28] An important breakthrough in clinical trial design followed from the shortages of a new drug, streptomycin, shortly after the war.

Following war trials of penicillin, British epidemiologist and biostatistician, A. Bradford Hill, was faced with the task of testing a promising antibiotic, streptomycin, against tuberculosis. Researchers in the United States studying the same drug had ample supplies and led to more effective treatment for patient subjects but produced less conclusive clinical trial data.[29] Hill and his colleagues, however, were faced with a severe shortage of the streptomycin drug they were studying. In post-war Britain, the central government could not afford to purchase more of the streptomycin drug. Scarcity and expense, therefore, justified their decision to formally but randomly assign patients to control groups and treatment groups. This eliminated a well-known form of treatment 'bias' in which physicians are known to select their healthier patients for experimental treatment leaving sicker patients in the control group. Hill's study was a true randomized study. It was not, however, 'double blinded' – another way of ensuring the objectivity of a trial by neutralizing the power of 'suggestion.'

In a double-blind clinical drug study, trials are designed in such a way that neither the patient nor the researcher knows who is receiving the treatment drug.[30] In Hill's study, streptomycin required injection, and the researchers did not wish to use inert injections. However, the lack of true double-blinding had little impact on the results,

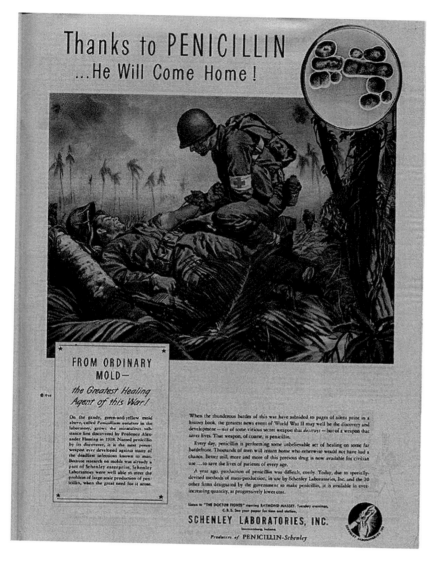

Following war trials of penicillin, British epidemiologist and biostatistician, A. Bradford Hill, was faced with the task of testing a promising antibiotic, streptomycin, against tuberculosis.

since Hill was able to show conclusively that streptomycin could cure tuberculosis. When the results of his study were published in 1948, Hill's use of concurrent controls (randomized, controlled) was praised as having ushered in "a new era of medicine."[31]

Hill and his North American colleagues, including Harry Gold at the Cornell Medical School, began to map out general criteria for drug testing and specify stages through which drug development should proceed. Patients were to be selected through formal criteria and then randomly separated into treatment and control groups; trials were to be double-blinded and employ objective diagnostic technologies; and drug doses were to be administered according to a fixed schedule, while patient observations were to be charted at uniform intervals. Their success set the stage for the subsequent development of more sophisticated clinical trial designs while professional collaborations allowed statisticians to increasingly dominate the conduct of clinical trials in the U.S.[32] Nonetheless, one expert estimated in 1951 that 45% of clinical trials had no control groups.[33]

After WWII, medical research increased exponentially in the United States. In 1950, funding for medical and scientific research was $161 million dollars. By 1968, this figure had grown to over $2.5 billion.[34] National Institutes of Health (NIH) opened its Clinical Center in Bethesda, MD as a research hospital in 1952, and NIH's extramural, peer-reviewed research grant system soon supported biomedical and clinical research projects at institutions around the country. Centrally planned clinical research projects, including cooperative trials, were soon eclipsed as grants supported the work of individual medical investigators, many of whom designed and conducted their own clinical trials in collaboration with other colleagues.

Ethical concerns about the protection of research subjects further complicated clinical trial design, post-war, particularly following reports of the gross medical abuses carried out on Nazi prisoners of war.[35] Ethical debates over methodology often centered around questions concerning when it was appropriate to use placebo controlled trials and when it was preferable to compare active treatments in evaluating new therapies. The NIH Clinical Center adopted a policy that placed much of the responsibility for safeguarding human subjects of biomedical research with principal investigators. Research involving normal human volunteers was to be formally reviewed by panels of scientists, but there was virtually no discussion about any potential role for the federal government in regulating medical research. Meanwhile, both NIH and FDA gave clinical investigators wide latitude in the pursuit of their research objectives.[36]

Sulfa drugs and antibiotics, among other therapies for acute diseases, had provided important experience in evaluating new drugs, but increasingly after WWII, investigators and regulatory officials began to rely on increasingly sophisticated trial designs to study effectiveness in whole new classes of drugs for chronic, rather than acute conditions. Blood pressure and anti-arrhythmic drugs (1950s/60s), drugs for tuberculosis, cancer, heart disease, and the oral contraceptives (1960) were all approved using new and increasingly advanced trial methodology involving assessment of data from sometimes tens of thousands of patients. Statisticians insisted on uniform selection criteria for patients in clinical trials, separate treatment and control groups, uniform dosing regimens, and utilized objective evidence from laboratory tests such as blood and urine tests made both before and after treatment. With the aid of a new science of biostatistics, both regulators and regulated industry began to understand, appreciate, and interpret many nuanced components of trial design and their effect on the interpretation of data.[37] Although several kinds of randomized controlled trial methodologies can be useful to researchers and regulators, ultimately, it was the randomized, double-blinded, placebo controlled experiment which became the standard by which most other experimental methods were judged, and it has often subsequently been referred to as the 'gold' standard for clinical trial methodology. In situations in which using a placebo seemed unethical, positive (treatment) groups rather than placebo groups were employed and regulators had to learn how to interpret the data stemming from these trials as well, a formidable problem in many cases.[38]

The Kefauver hearings and drug critics

In the early 1950s the AMA discontinued many of its drug study activities. It closed its microbiological laboratory used to test new drugs (successor to the Chemical Laboratory) and discontinued its Seal of Acceptance program. Since only drugs that had the Seal could advertise in the pages of AMA periodicals, the discontinuation of this program opened the door for an explosion of advertising (and advertising revenue) in JAMA and other AMA publications. AMA discontinued its inspection of drug plants, its efforts to exert some control over generic drug names, and even a campaign it had instituted to explain and encourage physicians to prescribe using generic names rather than brand names.[39] In their place, the AMA initiated a registry for reporting adverse drug reactions, although it had no mechanism to enforce data collection.[40]

Beginning in 1958, hearings on the drug industry … focused unanticipated attention on the quality of drug company sponsored clinical drug research.

Beginning in 1958, hearings on the drug industry held by Senator Estes Kefauver (Democrat- Tennessee) focused unanticipated attention on the quality of drug company sponsored clinical drug research. In particular, the hearings drew attention to the poor state of clinical trial research as it had been conducted (or failed to be conducted) under the 1938 statute. Kefauver announced his hearings on the drug industry – its products and its profitability – after he and his staff had obtained evidence documenting the high markups and exorbitant profit margins that had become evident on prescription drugs, beginning with antibiotics. Yet the hearings soon turned to other topics as the industry tried to defend its profits by asserting the high cost of research, including the costs of conducting clinical trials. As popular with consumers as they proved unpopular with the pharmaceutical industry, these hearings generated important evidence documenting the frequently sorry state of drug testing and advertising as well as the competitive pressures within the industry that supported such practices. Able testimony was offered documenting many poor clinical studies done in support of the marketing of many mediocre drugs. Dr. Louis Lasagna, an expert in clinical pharmacology, testified that it was "shocking that experimental drugs are subject to no FDA regulation of any sort before patients receive them. …It is reprehensible for man to be the first experimental animal on which toxicity tests are done, simply because bypassing toxicity tests in laboratory animals saves time and money."[41] At one point in the hearings a former medical director at Squibb testified that the industry was always pointing out the high costs of research and the fact that so many products failed in the course of research to justify its markups and profit margins. "This," he agreed, "was true, since it is the very essence of research." The problem, he quipped, lay in the fact that "they market so many of their failures."[42] Most new drug products, experts testified, were not improvements over old ones, and most were marketed before clinical studies were published. Many new drugs, in fact, were combinations of older drugs, with or without modification, which gained extended patent life (and profitability) in combination.

Years later, FDA's Chief Counsel William Goodrich recalled that during the Kefauver hearings the pharmaceutical industry, "stepped right into the bear trap" when it tried to defend itself by touting the high costs of research and development for new drugs. (See box on page 37).

By the 1960s, following another drug crisis in 1962, there was a growing recognition of the importance of clinical trials in new drug development as well as in clinical medicine. Pharmacologists and medical researchers as well as officials at government agencies such as the Veteran's Administration and the National Institutes of Health knew more about the conduct of good clinical trials than did the FDA at that time. This changed rapidly, however, beginning with a drug crisis in 1962. Following a pattern first seen in the elixir sulfanilamide crisis, which led to changes in U.S. drug regulation in 1938, a similar crisis in 1962 spurred even more widespread changes, both in the U.S. and around the world. In 1961, a popular drug in Europe, a hypnotic known as thalidomide, was discovered to cause severe birth defects and even death in babies when their mothers took the drug early in their pregnancies. Because of the concerns of FDA drug reviewer Dr. Frances Kelsey, the drug was never approved for sale in the U.S. Nonetheless, the drug sponsor had sent samples of the drug to thousands of U.S. doctors who gave the samples to their patients without telling them that the drug was an experimental one, making their patients the unwitting subjects of human drug experimentation. It is believed that there were more than a dozen thalidomide babies born in the United States as a result of this unauthorized "sample" program. As a result of the worldwide thalidomide disaster, countries around the world, including the United States, updated their drug regulatory systems and statutes. "In next to no time," recalled Frances Kelsey, "the fighting over the new drug laws that had been going on for five or six years suddenly melted away, and the 1962 amendments were passed almost immediately and unanimously."[44]

Arguments regarding the high costs of research

That just focused attention on these various phases of new drug development and promotion…first of all, was it really all that expensive? Were they really doing all that kind of research? And anyone who had looked at any of the New Drug Applications knew, as I knew, that that was all baloney, and what they were saying to us in those early days was essentially a bunch of testimonials. The way drugs were investigated–a physician from the company would go out in the community with some samples and say to the doctor, "I've got this new drug for so-and-so. Here's some samples. Try it out and let us know how you like it." And they would get back a letter from him: "I tried it out on eight patients and they all got along fine." That's the kind of stuff that was coming in for the science. Of course, that was completely unsatisfactory, and as soon as people focused on that, that raised the problem.[43]

The IND process and clinical trial regulation

Prior to the law's final passage, regulations began to address known problems in the use of clinical trials by the drug industry, indicating that FDA felt more confident in its authority to regulate them, even under the old 1938 statute.[45] New regulations prohibited testing a drug in humans until preclinical studies could predict that the drug could be given safely to people.[46] The 1962 [Kefauver-Harris] Drug Amendments and the 1963 investigational drug regulations themselves introduced many new procedures that strengthened control over investigational new drugs in the United States.[47] One of the most significant was a system of pre-clinical trial notification and approval designed to provide enough information to regulators to demonstrate that it was safe to conduct clinical trials. Under this new system, company drug sponsors were required to file a "notice of claimed investigational exemption for a new drug." The "notice" was actually a package of materials that a company submitted to FDA for approval prior to starting human trials. The acronym IND (Investigational New Drug) was coined to parallel the acronym NDA (New Drug Application).[48] Technically, an IND is an exemption from the normal pre-marketing requirements for a new drug – namely, the submission and approval of an NDA.[49] An approved IND application allows investigators to proceed with new drug trials for a drug under development. The information collected under an IND may later become a part of an NDA submission if the systematic drug tests set up to test the drug are successful. INDs are also required when a sponsor wishes to restudy a previously approved drug in order to gather data in support of significant labeling changes, advertising changes, changes in route of administration or dose, or any other change that might alter the risk/benefit equation upon which the original approval was based. The IND regulations also led FDA to define more clearly through regulation the 'phase' process of drug testing involved in the regulatory approval of a new drug in the 1963 regulations.[50]

> The acronym IND (Investigational New Drug) was coined to parallel the acronym NDA (New Drug Application). Technically, an IND is an exemption from the normal pre-marketing requirements for a new drug – namely, the submission and approval of an NDA.

An IND submission

1. Alerts regulators to a sponsor's intent to begin clinical studies in the United States
2. Provides the preliminary animal toxicity data indicating it is reasonably safe to administer the drug to humans
3. Provides information about the manufacturing process for the new drug
4. Provides chemistry background material
5. Describes the initial clinical study being proposed, focusing on its safety measures (who is conducting the trials, their qualifications and facilities; and the type of study population involved – volunteers, sick patients, prisoners, women, men, children, etc.) and
6. Provides assurance than an IRB (Institutional Review Board) will approve the study protocol before the study begins.

In addition to the IND submission itself, every investigator participating in the study must sign a form, maintained by the sponsor, indicating their qualifications, the location of the research facility where the study will be conducted, and the name of the IRB responsible for reviewing and approving the study protocol. Investigators must sign commitments to:

1. Conduct the clinical study in accordance with the IRB approved protocol
2. Personally conduct or supervise the conduct of the investigation
3. Inform potential subjects that the drugs are being used for investigational purposes and
4. Report to the sponsor adverse events that occur in the course of the investigation.

Efficacy under the 1962 drug amendments

A new and key provision in the 1962 amendments was the requirement that, in addition to the pre-market demonstrations of safety already required under the 1938 Act, future new drugs would also have to be demonstrated "efficacious" prior to marketing. This provision required controlled trials that could indeed support claims of efficacy. The 60-day approval 'default' under the 1938

Act was removed. New drugs had to have positive and specific, and increasingly detailed approval from FDA to go to market and FDA was given the authority to set standards for every stage of drug testing from laboratory to clinic. In addition, FDA could require market withdrawals for the first time and establish 'Good Manufacturing Practices' (GMP's) to govern drug manufacturing.

In order to prevent another 'thalidomide disaster,' Congress inserted language in the 1962 Drug Amendments requiring that investigators maintain personal supervision over clinical investigations and agree not to give the drug to other investigators. Senator Jacob Javits (Democrat-New York) was particularly concerned about the fact that so many people had taken thalidomide without knowing that it was an experimental drug. Even many doctors that FDA had surveyed had been confused as to the status of the drug at the time they gave it to their patients.[51] Javits sponsored what became a very important provision of the law itself: the requirement that informed consent be obtained from all research study subjects so that patients would have to be specifically informed if a drug they were being given or prescribed was 'experimental,' something that had not happened in the case of thalidomide.

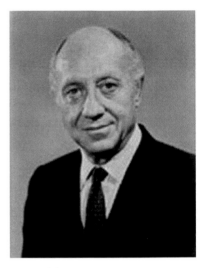

Senator Jacob Javits was particularly concerned about the fact that so many people had taken thalidomide without knowing that it was an experimental drug.

The legal language employed in the statute, which laid out the criteria that would be used in assessing efficacy in support of a new drug approval, was not particularly stringent. The law required that there be "substantial evidence" that the drug "will have the effect it purports or is represented to have under the conditions of use prescribed, recommended, or suggested in the proposed labeling." Lawyers have concluded that Congress could have established a more stringent drug approval process simply by using stronger legal terminology. The fact that terms such as "preponderance of evidence" or "evidence beyond a reasonable doubt" were not used indicates that Congress did not intend to set the bar for efficacious new drug approvals too high.[52] New drugs did not have to be superior to other drugs on the market nor did "substantial evidence" mean evidence "so strong as to convince everyone."[53]

The strength in the statutory language, however, came not from the evidentiary requirements but from a last minute-compromise over study methods.[54] Sponsors were only required to provide "substantial evidence" of effectiveness, but that evidence had to be based on "adequate and well-controlled studies," i.e. clinical trials. Without defining either "adequate" or "well-controlled," the law paved the way for experts in the field to establish the criteria that would define both terms under the new statute. Although the law did not define a well-controlled study, testimony before Congress made it clear that it included, as a minimum, the use of control groups, random allocation of patients to control and therapeutic groups, and techniques to minimize bias including standardized criteria for judging effectiveness.[55] A poorly designed trial, it was argued, not only wasted resources, but it unnecessarily put patients at risk.

Clinical trial regulations of 1970 and the DESI process

Over the next eight years FDA worked diligently to implement the 1962 drug amendments. In the early years after passage of the 1962 amendments, sponsors were more or less 'on their own' with little guidance from FDA about what would be acceptable except in the form of an NDA non-approval letter which did explain why the sponsors' submission was considered inadequate. Concerns that FDA might become overly 'vested' in the development of a commercial drug product led to an abundance of caution in agency/sponsor interactions. According to one official, "There was, in fact, explicit concern that too much participation by FDA staff in the development process would leave the Agency unable to be properly neutral and analytical when the resulting data were submitted as part of an NDA."[56] Over the years, however, as Robert Temple notes, FDA has become increasingly involved in the development of specific drug products including the design of clinical trials, "reflecting the view that the public, the industry, and the FDA are poorly served by drug development efforts that are poorly designed or inadequate and that therefore waste resources and delay availability of therapy."[57] In the late twentieth century, Congress itself has even begun mandating meetings between regulators and industry concerning the design and conduct of clinical trials deemed particularly important for any of a number of reasons.[58]

Regulatory officials soon began to receive an invaluable education in the conduct of clinical trials as a result of the agency's Drug Efficacy Study (DES). The 1962 Drug Amendments required FDA to re-review all drugs that had been approved under the 1938 Food, Drug, and Cosmetic Act (1938-1962) on the basis of safety alone, this time looking for evidence of efficacy. Industry objected to submitting pre-1962 drug records for review to FDA itself, and in 1966, FDA contracted with the National Research Council of the National Academy of Sciences to perform the review.[59] Thirty panels of experts reviewed specific drug categories using evidence from obtained from FDA, the drug's manufacturer, scientific literature, and the personal expertise of the panel members themselves. Their ratings on each claim for a drug fell into six categories:

> **The 1962 Drug Amendments required FDA to re-review all drugs that had been approved under the 1938 Food, Drug, and Cosmetic Act (1938-1962) on the basis of safety alone, this time looking for evidence of efficacy.**

1. Effective
2. Probably effective
3. Possibly effective
4. Ineffective
5. Effective but, and
6. Ineffective as a fixed combination (combination drugs for which there was no substantial reason to believe that each ingredient adds to the effectiveness of the combination.).[60]

FDA was challenged to devise a method by which those drugs ruled ineffective could be legally removed from the market along with other 'me-too' drugs – drugs with the same essential ingredient profile. FDA's initial legal efforts to remove bioflavonoid drugs and an UpJohn fixed combination drug called Panalba were enjoined by the courts.[61] Faced with the prospect of conducting formal administrative hearings on every drug it proposed to have removed from the market, the agency changed its approach, led by FDA's Director of the Bureau of Medicine (and later Commissioner) Dr. Herbert Ley. Ley supported the drafting, publication and implementation of regulations defining "substantial evidence" leading to a showing of effectiveness under the 1962 Amendments.

These "evidence rules" had two separate components but companies wishing an administrative hearing on the proposed withdrawal of their pre-1962 drug would have to meet both criteria:

1. The first formally specified the scientific content of "adequate and well-controlled clinical investigations, including clinical investigations, by experts qualified by scientific training and experience to evaluate the effectiveness of the drug involved," under the 1962 statute. Well-controlled trials did not have to be placebo controlled-- they could have active controls, or even historical controls-- but the regulations stated clearly that, "uncontrolled studies are not acceptable evidence to support claims of effectiveness."[62] No hearing would be granted unless there was a "reasonable likelihood" that such evidence would be forthcoming.[63]

2. The second required the submission of positive results from at least two clinical studies in order to escape an automatic withdrawal of approval for the drug without a hearing.[64] The courts upheld the agency's new approach and according to Peter Barton Hutt, FDA's Chief Counsel from 1971-1975, no hearings were deemed necessary.

By the end of 1971, FDA had disposed of dozens of requests for hearings on the revocation of NDA's. In no instance had it determined that a manufacturer's supporting data were sufficient to justify a hearing. One explanation of this striking consistency is that the agency's substantial evidence regulations embodied requirements for clinical investigations that few pre-1962 studies could meet. The drugs it initially selected for withdrawal, those evaluated by the NAS-NRC as "ineffective" also presented the easiest targets. But it was becoming obvious that a manufacturer would have to make an overwhelming showing to persuade FDA to expend the time and resources that even one hearing would require.[65]

> By the end of 1971, FDA had disposed of dozens of requests for hearings on the revocation of NDA's.

The results of the DES study led to recommendations soon implemented through the Drug Efficacy Study Implementation (DESI), which removed over 1000 ineffective drugs and drug combinations from the marketplace. As part of this process, FDA drug reviewers themselves published hundreds of critiques of the clinical studies that had been submitted for approved new drugs in support of the safety requirements mandated in the 1938 statute. Most of these old studies, recalled Robert Temple, who began work at FDA in 1972, were "inadequate beyond belief." As late as the 1960s and early 1970s he notes, "You would be horrified [at the clinical trial data submitted to the agency]. There was often no protocol at all. There was almost never a statistical plan. Sequential analyses were unheard of. It was a very different world."[66]

Positive changes in clinical trial methodology, however, soon began to be evident in new NDA and ANDA submissions. "Everyone," notes Temple, "came to believe that trials should have a prospectively defined and identified endpoint, a real hypothesis and an actual analytical plan." An international, professional organization, the Society for Clinical Trials, was organized in 1978 and began to develop and discuss clinical trial design and the analysis of clinical trials in government as well as industry sponsored clinical trial research. FDA assisted the drug industry during the late 1970s, by collaborating with external advisory committees and conducting FDA-industry workshops in support of the development of nearly 30 drug class clinical guidelines which described in detail the study designs and expected data required for particular therapeutic classes such as drugs for ulcer disease, depression, or angina.

> An international, professional organization, the Society for Clinical Trials, was organized in 1978 and began to develop and discuss clinical trial design and the analysis of clinical trials ...

During the AIDS epidemic of the 1980s, regulators were again pushed to consider the essential requirements of a meaningful clinical trial. FDA had created a special class of investigations known as the "Treatment IND" in 1987 in which patients could receive an investigational drug outside the normal "blinded" research setting.[67] Although data from patients under this protocol was still collected, the program was not especially conducive to the treatment of large numbers of patients, especially those desperately sick patients who pushed for access to drugs at their earliest stages of development.[68]

In 1985 regulations recognized what had already become a central tenet of modern drug evaluation by formalizing the requirement that approvals be based on an "integrated summary of all available information about the safety of a drug product."[69] Congress itself mandated in 1988 that each AIDS drug IND must be publicly disclosed in a computer-accessible data base to facilitate access by patients with AIDS, and formally recognized the importance of FDA's Treatment IND program in support of AIDS patients.[70] Although some AIDS organizations requested agency support of 'open clinicals' in which a drug sponsor could allow any patient access to ongoing trials with the support of their physicians, FDA refused to allow such easy access. "The more open-ended the design of a clinical trial," noted agency officials, "the less likely the chance the trial will provide answers."[71] Between 1990 and 1992 guidelines were proposed and negotiated, and regulations finally approved by FDA establishing a "parallel track approval" process in which special categories of drugs would be expedited during the review process and a wider group of patients would have access to the drug than under normal procedures.[72]

Beginning in the mid 1980s, FDA has focused on improving the analysis of data from clinical trials. One lesson learned from the AIDS epidemic and the concomitant development of clinical trials necessary to test drug products for its treatment is the scientific utility of surrogate endpoints in certain circumstances. Some of this data analysis has been motivated by sponsors' interest in presenting evidence of clinical effectiveness through measurements of biomarkers and evaluation of "surrogate endpoints." Surrogate endpoints measure outcomes that are not clinically valuable by themselves (lowered cholesterol, blood pressure, elevated T-cell counts) but are thought to correspond with improved clinical outcomes (decreased heart disease or stroke, fewer opportunistic infections for AIDS patients). FDA approved the first statin drug, for example, in 1987, based on the surrogate of lowering blood cholesterol.[73] FDA is cautious, however, in accepting surrogates and usually requires continued post-market study to verify and describe continued clinical benefits. In 1992, new regulations for the accelerated approval of new drugs gave the agency explicit authority to rely on a surrogate marker.[74]

> In 1994, FDA made changes in its policies designed to facilitate women's participation in the earliest phases of clinical drug trials.

In 1994, FDA made changes in its policies designed to facilitate women's participation in the earliest phases of clinical drug trials.[75] Most recently, FDA has issued guidelines promoting greater study and better analysis of patient subgroups including drugs in the elderly, separate analysis of trial data for both genders, and pediatric studies as well as dose-response information.[76]

The future

In an era in which health care costs are rising at rates far higher than the rate of inflation and the nation faces the challenge of promoting the health of the 'boomer' generation during its retirement years, there have been cries for more comparative drug studies, in part to help contain drug costs. Greater knowledge of genetic science and the ability to conduct more nuanced analyses of drug trial data, including retrospective meta-analyses, have also helped fuel optimism over the future of personalized medicine. In the past the drug industry has concentrated on developing so called 'block-buster' drugs. The large scale, randomized clinical trial has been critical in demonstrating the safety and efficacy of these drugs. Many, however, are predicting that the future of medicine points toward developing drugs and diagnostics to treat sub-sets of patients who may respond to one treatment but not another because of genetic and other factors. This has led many to speculate on the future of randomized trials. "The randomized clinical trial is excellent methodology if you want to understand, *on average*, whether one treatment is better than another treatment," notes John Bridges, assistant professor at Johns Hopkins School of Public Health, "but if we think about a distribution of outcomes, no single person in the health care system is the average."[77] Personalized medicine presents challenges of its own, including increased costs for researchers testing drugs and patients taking them. It seems more likely that better analysis of clinical trial data, already being encouraged by the FDA, and pursued by both researchers and drug sponsors as the first step towards a more personalized perspective on drug development, will be an integral part of the evolution of personalized medicine, while continuing to add to our overall knowledge of the safety and effectiveness profiles of medicines and therapeutics already on the market. The randomized clinical trial is unlikely, in either scenario, to go the way of the dinosaur.

References

1. 5600 Fishers Lane, room 12-69, Rockville, MD 20857. Suzanne.Junod@fda.hhs.gov.

2. Affadavit of William Thomas Beaver, M.D. in the case of Pharmaceutical Manufacturers Association v. Robert H. Finch and Herbert Ley, Civil Action No. 3797, United States District Court for the District of Columbia

3. Harry Marks *The Progress of Experiment: Science and Therapeutic Reform in the United States, 1900-1990* (Cambridge: Cambridge University Press, 1997). Hereafter referred to as Marks, *Progress*

4. The 1938 Act recognized the purity standards published by the U.S.P. and the National Formulary. The U.S.P under the new law was responsible for all packaging and labeling standards while FDA enforced these standards. See Arthur Daemmrich, "Pharmacovigilance and the Missing Denominator: The Changing Context of Pharmaceutical Risk Mitigation, *Pharmacy in History* 49:2 (2007), p. 64.

5. John P. Bull, "The Historical Development of Clinical Therapeutic Trials," *Journal of Chronic Diseases* 10:3 (1959), p. 219.

6. *Ibid.*

7. Bull, p. 228.

8. Geoffrey Edsall, "A Positive Approach to the Problem of Human Experimentation," in Experimentation, p. 279.

9. Bob Temple, "Government Viewpoint of Clinical Trials," *Drug Information Journal* 82: January/June (1981), p. 10.

10. Marks, *Progress*, p. 12.

11. Susan Lederer, *Subjected to Science: Human Experimentation in America Before the Second World War* (Baltimore: Johns Hopkins, 1995), p. xiv.

12. *Ibid,* p. 19.

13. Arthur Daemmrich, "Pharmacovigilance and the Missing Denominator," p. 64.

14. Harry F. Dowling, "The Emergence of the Cooperative Clinical Trial," *Transactions and Studies of the College of Physicians of Philadelphia* 43 (1975), pp. 20-29. Marks, *Progress*, p. 53-54.

15. *Brown v. Hughes* (94 Colo. 295, 30 P. 2d 259 (1934). Ironically, at this time, many if not most of these "accepted" clinical practices were not based upon rigorous scientific study.

16. *Fortner v. Koch* (272 Mich. 273; 261 NW 762 (1935) as commented on by William J. Curran, "Governmental Regulation of the Use of Human Subjects in Medical Research: The Approach of Two Federal Agencies," in *Experimentation with Human Subjects,* ed. Paul A. Freund, pp. 402-455. Hereafter cited as *Experimentation.*

17. 35 Fed. Reg. 7250 (May 8, 1970). The 1970 regulations recognized comparative evidence from no-treatment and treatment groups, placebo controlled trials, active treatment trials (comparing treatments), and historical controls.

18. Initial regulations under the 1938 Act (issued December 28, 1938), required the person who introduced an investigational new drug into interstate commerce to obtain from the expert (qualified by scientific training and experience to investigate the safety of drugs, i.e. the clinical investigator) "a signed statement . . . that he has adequate facilities for the investigation to be conducted by him and that such drug

will be used solely by him or under his direction for the investigation." This was, of course, unless or until an NDA was approved by FDA.

19. Robert Temple, "Development of Drug Law, Regulations, and Guidance in the U.S," Principles of Pharmacy (1994), p. 1643.

20. Marks, *Progress,* p. 72.

21. Dowling, "The Emergence of the Cooperative Clinical Trial," p. 25-29.

22. See, for example, Suzanne Junod and Lara Marks, "Women's Trials: The Approval of the First Oral Contraceptive Pill in the United States and Great Britain," *Journal of the History of Medicine and Allied Sciences,* 57: 2 (April 2002), pp. 117-160.

23. 52 Stat. 1040, 21 U.S.C. June 25, 1938.

24. Arthur Daemmrich, "Pharmacovigilance and the Missing Denominator," p. 64.

25. The reference to investigational drugs under section 355(i) of the 1938 Act was brief. "The Secretary shall promulgate regulations for exempting from the operation of this section drugs intended solely for investigational use by experts qualified by scientific training and experience to investigate the safety of drugs." Food, Drug, and Cosmetic Act, 52 Stat. 1040 (75th Cong. 3d Sess (1938)).

26. Arthur A. Daemmrich, *Pharmacopolitics: Drug Regulation in the United States and Germany* (Chapel Hill: University of North Carolina Press, 2004), p. 24. Hereafter cited as Daemmich, *Drug Regulation.*

27. Winkle, Harwick, Calvery, and Smith, "Laboratory and Clinical Appraisal of New Drugs," JAMA 126 (1944), 956-61.

28. Daemmrich, p. 51.

29. Dowling, "The Emergence of the Cooperative Clinical Trial," p. 24.

30. Ibid. p. 52.

31. Silverman and Chalmers, "Sir Austin Bradford Hill," p. 102.

32. Daemmrich, p. 52.

33. Ross, "Use of Controls in Medical Research," *JAMA* 145 (1951), pp. 72-75.

34. Curran, *Experimentation,* p. 402.

35. At the 1946 Nuremberg trial of 23 Nazi medical professionals, only a handful of victims survived to confront their torturers, out of hundreds of thousands of prisoners. The defendants were charged with offenses ranging from subjecting test subjects to extremes of altitude and temperature to using them as human cultures to test vaccines for typhus and malaria. In light of the testimony, an international code of ethics to protect all subjects of human research was written and adopted by most medical researchers in countries worldwide. The Nuremberg Code accepted and codified ethical standards which the 23 defendants had grossly violated, and thus became the first internationally recognized code of medical research ethics. Its stated goal was not merely to "prevent experimental abominations in the future but to increase the protection of the rights and welfare of human subjects everywhere by clarifying the standards of integrity that constrain the pursuit of knowledge." The first principle of the Nuremberg Code stressed the importance of obtaining "informed consent" from research subjects. The code also emphasized that human studies should not be random or unnecessary, that animal studies should be undertaken before human studies, and that surveys of the natural histories of disease should be undertaken before subjecting human subjects to laboratory-induced disease.

36. Curran, *Experimentation,* p. 508. Research involving normal human volunteers was to be formally reviewed by panels of scientists.

37. Bradford Hill, "Medical Ethics and Controlled Trials" British Medical Journal 1 (April 20, 1963), pp. 1043-49.

38. Susan Ellenberg and Robert Temple, "Placebo Controlled Trials and Active-Control Trials in the Evaluation of New Treatments," *Annals of Internal Medicine* 133:6 (Sept. 19, 2000), pp. 455-470; ICH E-10 (Choice of Control Group and Related Issues in Clinical Trials) @http://inside.fda.gov/portal/page?_pageid=197,726738&_dad=portal&_schema=PORTAL (site last visited 10/17/07). Robert Temple, "Government Viewpoint of Clinical Trials, *Drug Information Journal* 82 (1981), pp. 10-17.

39. Richard Harris, *The Real Voice* (New York: The McMillan Company, 1964), p. 126.

40. Daemmrich, "Pharmacovigilance and the Missing Denominator," p. 64-65.

41. 'Statement on S 1552" Louis Lasagna, Drug Industry Anti-Trust Act, p. 1083.

42. Ibid. p. 78-79.

43. Oral History Interview with William Goodrich, former FDA-er interviewed in 1986, FDA History website, www.fda.gov/oc/history/default.htm. Last visited 10/22/07.

44. Frances Kelsey, Autobiographical Reflections, p. 71. FDA History Office.

45. Notice of Proposed Rulemaking, 27 Fed Reg 7990 (August 10, 1962).

46. Specifically, the requirement was that before clinical testing could proceed, drug sponsors had to submit "reports of pre-clinical tests (including tests on animals) of such drug adequate to justify proposed clinical testing." Notice of Proposed Rulemaking, 27 Fed Reg 7990 (August 10, 1962).

47. 76 Stat.780 (October 10, 1962) PL 87-781; 28 Fed. Reg. 179 (January 8, 1963); 28 Fed. Reg. 5048 (May 20, 1963); 28 Fed. Reg. 10972 (October 11, 1963).

48. Frances Kelsey, Autobiographical Reflections, p. 71. FDA History Office.

49. Robert Temple, "Development of Drug Law, Regulations and Guidance in the U.S." chapter 113 Principles of Pharmacology, pp. 1643-1664 (1994), p. 1644.

50. 28 FR 179 (January 8, 1963) 130.3 (a)(10). See also, Robert Temple, "Current definitions of phases of investigation and the role of the FDA in the conduct of clinical trials" American Heart Journal 139: 2000: S133-S135.

Clinical trials today are referred to by regulators, clinicians, and investigators as being in or having completed Phase I, Phase II, Phase III, and even Phase IV trials (post-marketing studies). There may be considerable overlap, but in general, Phase I study provides the first human studies of a new drug either in patients or in human volunteers. Although the number of participants can vary, Phase I trials usually involve twenty to eighty people. These early trials can provide early evidence of effectiveness, but they are designed to furnish greater understanding of the experimental drug's safety including side effects in relation to drug dose. Ideally, a Phase I study should be designed to provide enough information about the drug to design a well-controlled Phase II study.

A Phase II study is the first controlled clinical study to evaluate the effectiveness of a drug for a specific therapeutic use in patients. It is a well controlled, closely monitored study, usually with no more than a few hundred patients. Such studies look at the effects of treatment on symptoms or on a surrogate for a clinical outcome (i.e. lowered blood pressure, decreased viral load, etc.). Ideally such studies are double-blind placebo-controlled investigations in which patients are randomly assigned to a drug treatment group or a placebo group and neither the patient nor the investigator knows, until the end of the trial, which option the patient received. Phase II studies are also the first to consider the risk of a drug's side effects.

Phase III drug trials are reserved for experimental drugs which have shown at least some evidence of effectiveness in previous trials. They involve large numbers of patients (several hundred to several thousand) and are designed to gather enough information on safety and effectiveness to allow an adequate assessment of a risk/benefit ratio for the study drug as well as for the preparation of material for physician's labeling. They also use a broader patient population and can be designed to gather longer term safety and effectiveness data as well as data to establish optimum drug dosing. Phase III trials also typically have a data monitoring committee overseeing the collection of data during the trials.

51. Frances Kelsey, "Autobiographical Reflections," p. 73. FDA History Office.

52. "In American legal terms, "substantial evidence" is not a high standard; indeed, it has been described by a former FDA chief counsel as somewhere between a "scintilla and a preponderance." *Ibid*.

53. Robert Temple, "Development of Drug Law, Regulations and Guidance in the U.S," p. 1644.

54. Harris, *The Real Voice* (New York: McMillan Press, 1964), pp. 204-205. Harris' account of the final negotiations over the 1962 Amendments makes it clear that industry did not fully appreciate the significance of the phrase "adequate and well-controlled investigations" at the time it agreed to it. Counsel for the Department of Health, Education, and Welfare immediately grasped the significance and remarked that [the language adopted] "gives us all kinds of power – especially the word 'adequate' – to make sure that drugs do what is claimed for them."

55. Animal studies were not mandated under the new law, but within a few years following passage of the 1962 amendments, a fairly standardized set of animal toxicology studies to precede and support human trials was in place. By the 1970s a drug for chronic use would generally be required to be tested in two animal species for the full lifetime of the animal at the maximum tolerated dose. Temple, *Principles,* p. 1646. New York Academy of Medicine: Committee on Public Health, "The importance of clinical testing in determining the efficacy and safety of drugs," *Bull. N.Y. Acad. Med.* 38: 415-439, 1962.

56. Robert Temple, "Development of Drug Law, Regulations, and Guidance in the U.S., in *Principles of Pharmacology,* 1994, p. 1646.

57. Ibid., p. 1647.

58. During the mid-1970s, allegations of a "drug lag" in the approval of new drugs made officials more willing to meet with sponsors at the end of Phase 2 drug testing. In Congress enacted the Orphan Drugs Act to encourage the development of drugs to treat rare diseases. Sponsors of orphan drugs were offered the right to ask for FDA assistance in their research planning. In 1987, revised IND regulations offered more meetings to sponsors, though "primarily" for IND's involving NME's or major new uses of marketed drugs. Requests for meetings, the regulations stated, would be honored "to the extent that FDA's resources permit." In 1988 regulations designed to facilitate development of drugs for life-threatening or debilitating diseases also allowed sponsors of such drugs to request earlier meetings with regulators.

59. 31 Fed. Reg. 9425 (July 9, 1966) and 31 Fed. Reg. 13014 (October 6, 1966).

60. Richard A. Merrill and Peter Barton Hutt, *Food and Drug Law: Casebook and Materials* (Mineola: Foundation Press, 1980), p. 373.

61. Panalba established the legal validity underlying FDA's current rules requiring a combination drug to show that the combination product is more effective than each component used separately.

62. 34 Fed Reg 14596 (September 19, 1969), 130.12 (a)(5) and (7)(b)(iii).

63. Oral History Interview, William Goodrich, FDA History website, www.fda.gov/oc/history/default.htm. "Having talked about the adequate and well-controlled clinical study regulations, I want to be sure I attribute to Herb Ley full credit for that. . . . it was Herb Ley who really put that thing through and gave it some scientific stature that it otherwise wouldn't have had. Paradoxically, Herb was doing this, which is one of the greatest things that ever happened to Food and Drug, yet at the same time he was losing his job over cyclamates."

64. 34 Fed. Reg. 14596 (September 19, 1969).

65. Merrill and Hutt, *Casebook,* p. 375.

66. Robert Temple, "How FDA Currently Makes Decisions on Clinical Studies," *Clinical Trials* 2 (2005), p. 276.

67. Robert Temple makes the point that the impetus for the development of the Treatment IND was "perceived as a response to AIDS, but its origins go back to around 1980 before HIV was identified." Robert Temple, "Development of Drug Law, Regulations and Guidance in the U.S.," p. 1660.

68. James T. O'Reilly, *Food and Drug Administration* (New York: McGraw Hill, 1993), p. 13-87.

69. According to Robert Temple, "the idea that safety data should be looked at all together, as opposed to study-by-study, is a relatively recent insight." Temple, "Drug Law Development," p. 1649.

70. 102 Stat 3066 (1988). Frank Young, "New Information Available About AIDS Treatments," *FDA Consumer* 23:6 (1989).

71. FDA Talk Paper T-88-74, FDA Responds to ACT-UP Demands (October 5, 1988).

72. Comment, "Prescription Drug Approval and Terminal Diseases: Desparate Times Require Desparate Measures, 44 *Vanderbilt Law Review* (1991), p. 925. Kiser, "Legal Issues Raised by Expedited Approval of and Expedited Access to Experimental AIDS Treatments, *Food, Drug, and Cosmetic Law Journal* 45 (1990), p. 363.

73. Suzanne Junod, "Statins: A Success Story Involving FDA, Academia, and Industry," FDLI *Update* (March/April 2007), p. 41.

74. Temple, "Drug Law Development," p. 1656.

75. Ruth Merkatz and Suzanne Junod, "Historical Background of Changes in FDA Policy on the Study and Evaluation of Drugs in Women," *Academic Medicine* 69:9 (1994), 703-707.

76. Temple, "Development of Drug Law, Regulations and Guidance in the U.S.", p. 1646.

77. "Is Comparative Effectiveness Antithetical to Personalized Medicine," RPM Report 2:9 (September 2007).

Chapter 3

The business of successful clinical drug development

James E. McClurg, Ph.D., Senior Vice President, Chief Scientific Officer, MDS Pharma Services

Todd Johnson, M.D., Senior Vice President, Strategy and Corporate Development, MDS Pharma Services

Integration of clinical care and clinical research to manage health care and drug development in the same process.

Risk

Drug discovery and development is a risky business. Bringing a new drug to market – from concept in discovery, through preclinical, early clinical (Phase I), and late clinical research (Phases II-IV) to regulatory approval – requires a significant commitment of time and money, often over eight years and often at a cost of $100 million or more. Along the way, drug candidates with less desirable traits are culled (despite the often significant investment made), leading to the industry's common philosophy of "fail early, fail cheap." The billions of dollars spent every year on 'attrited' molecules is an accepted risk of this business; on average only one of every 500 to 1000 drug candidates identified in the discovery laboratory enters clinical trials to be tested for 'clinical proof of concept' in humans[1]. Thereafter, additional tens or even hundreds of millions of dollars are invested in conducting the human clinical trials necessary to substantiate safety and efficacy claims for market approval. Approximately 8% of new drugs that enter clinical trials make it to the market, but this varies by therapeutic area. For example, an estimated 20% of cardiovascular drugs entering early clinical development have made it to the market, though that number can vary substantially (e.g., an average of 20% of cardiovascular drugs entering early clinical development attain regulatory approval, whereas only 5% of anti-cancer drugs and 8% of central nervous system (CNS) drugs will ever be marketed). To make matters worse, recent years have shown the risk and investment required for drug development is increasing due to falling research and development productivity.

> Drug discovery and development is a risky business.

Table 1: Number of compounds entering development phase (2000-2002). [2]

Preclinical	13
Phase I	9
Phase II	5
Phase III/file	2
Launch	1
Cumulative success	*8%*

This productivity decrease is occurring despite a rapidly expanding base of potential new targets for treating disease and quantum leaps in the numbers of compounds synthesized and screened using combinatorial chemistry and high-throughput methods. Since 1993, R&D spending has increased over threefold after inflation, while the numbers of new molecular entities approved by FDA has fallen from the 30 to 50 per year in the late 1990s to 15 to 25 in recent years.[3] The industry can expect big risks, declining development productivity, sustained healthcare needs and sizeable returns for those who successfully bring the right compounds to market.

> **The industry can expect big risks, declining development productivity, sustained healthcare needs and sizeable returns for those who successfully bring the right compounds to market.**

Costs

Drug development is a big business. Clinical development is the largest R&D segment in the industry, spending 37% of the total cost of a drug, and employing more than 50% of the R&D staff headcount. Research-based pharmaceutical companies in 2004 had more than 2,300 compounds in clinical development, spent 15.9% of their revenues ($39 billion) on R&D, and had a sales base of $244 billion. [2] Viewed another way, many research-based pharmaceutical companies are spending 16% of today's revenue to secure revenue growth on a five to seven year horizon, with 80-90% of that spending not ultimately directly linked to producing a marketed compound. In other words, the market is highly speculative with a long-term 'incubation period' before it can generate its sought-after market-driven return on investment.

Pfizer spent more on R&D than any company in any business in the world in 2006 ($8.18 billion), and seven of the top 20 globally ranked companies for R&D spending are pharmaceutical companies. Six of those seven show R&D spending growth over the prior year of 10% to $24 Billion. [4]

Cost estimates to get a new drug to the US market, fully capitalized and including cost of failures, ranges from $800 million to $1.7 billion.[2] Drug development is risky and expensive.

Managing risk

Given these brutal facts, reducing risk in drug development is a critical business need for those involved in pharmaceutical and biotechnology innovation. Seasoned and experienced planning reduces risk. How risk is viewed in drug development differs depending on which of several stakeholders you ask. For example, product managers and investors are focused toward development risk. Development risk depends not only on the financial resources available but on what expertise can be engaged in the development of a drug, the regulatory requirements involved, and what other expectations exist for the product (e.g., time required for development).

Investigators, the institutional review boards and drug regulatory bodies are concerned with risk to the patient. At the end of the day, marketing approval is based on an argument of risks-benefit or safety (injury) versus efficacy (improved health). A good clinical development and regulatory plan reflects the collective voices of the many stakeholders involved. An effectively designed and executed plan means that the drug product will "live or die" based on its inherent properties and not because of poor product development decisions, inadequate investment and planning or poor execution.

Research on R&D spending for pharmaceuticals, and results suggest little evidence that increasing R&D investment delivers increased performance results.

Research on R&D spending for pharmaceuticals, and results suggest little evidence that increasing R&D investment delivers increased performance results. The consulting firm Booz Allen Hamilton concludes, "It's the process not the pocketbook. Superior results seem to be a function of the quality of an organization's innovation process—the bets it makes and how it pursues them—rather than either the absolute or relative magnitude of its innovation spending.[5]

Effective clinical drug development has evolved into a well defined, linear process that proceeds through several high-level go/no go 'decision gates'.[6] These gates separate identifiable phases in clinical development and address specific major questions about the drug product as summarized in Table 2.

For a drug candidate to progress through one gate to the next phase, it must meet a set of criteria that have been previously agreed upon by the decision makers. It is a "go/no go" because the future product life of the drug hangs in the balance. Once the decision is made to progress a drug through a decision gate, the organization should be committed to spend even greater resources (money and scientists' time) to do the studies to address criteria for the next decision gate along the development path.

Table 2: Decision Gates in the Clinical Development Process

Decision Gate	Key Question	Source of Answers
Preclinical to First-in-Human (FIH)	Is drug safe enough to give to human subjects?	Preclinical pharmacology, safety and ADME studies. Adequate CMC.
FIH to Clinical Proof-of-Concept (PoC)	Is there evidence drug is working in humans as predicted from animal studies?	Phase I safety/tolerance and PK studies in healthy subjects Phase IIa study in small group of patients
PoC to End-of- Phase II Meeting	Does the drug perform well enough to proceed to Phase III studies?	Phase IIb studies looking at dose-response and duration-response, identification of non-responders, potential key drug-drug interactions
NDA/BLA approval	Is the drug safe and efficacious enough to be marketed?	Pivotal efficacy and long-term safety studies in targeted population Long term toxicology studies Technology transfer to scale up for commercial production
Life Cycle Management	Are there other indications or subpopulations that will improve drug sales?	Phase IV clinical studies to support additions or changes to the label, new indications or more efficient manufacturing methods.

Note: (ADME) Absorption, distribution, metabolism and excretion; (BLA) Biological License Application; (CMC) Chemistry Manufacturing and Controls; (NDA) New Drug Application;

(PK) Pharmacokinetic

Table 3: Drug Development Decision Analysis – Target Product Profile for Product "X"

	Human Safety	Dose-Response	PK/ADME	CMC	Regulatory
Best Achievable (*Enhance investment to assure timely completion*)	■ No treatment-related SAEs observed in Phase I/II studies ■ AEs <15% of subjects treated ■ No predicted drug-drug interactions	■ Therapeutic Index > 20 ■ Responders and non-responders can be clearly identified	■ Half-life supports once daily dosing ■ No effect of CYP inhibitors on clearance ■ AUC is proportional to dose ■ No food effect on bioavailability	■ Drug tablets stable for at least 1 year ■ Cost of goods for API < $5K/kg	■ Fast track review granted ■ Agreement at end-of-Phase II meeting with regulators on design and size of pivotal efficacy and safety studies to support therapeutic claim.
Base Case (*Invest in next phase*)	■ Treatment related SAEs < 0.5% ■ Overall AEs < 30% ■ Few predicted drug-drug interactions – can be managed with predictable dosing adjustments	■ Therapeutic Index > 10 ■ Advantage over current marketed product ■ Responders and non-responders can be clearly identified	■ Half-life supports once daily dosing ■ CYP inhibitors result in <30% increase in clearance ■ AUC is proportional to dose ■ Food decreases bio-availability <20%	■ Drug tablets stable for at least 6 mo ■ Cost of goods for API < $8K/kg	■ Agreement with regulators at end-of-phase II meeting on design and size of pivotal efficacy and safety studies to support therapeutic claim.
Minimum Required (*Proceed with caution*)	■ Treatment-related SAEs at higher exposures (risk can be mitigated with specific monitoring) ■ Overall AEs < 30% ■ Some manageable drug-drug interactions	■ Therapeutic Index > 5 ■ Equal to current marketed product	■ Half-life supports twice daily dosing ■ CYP inhibitors result in <50% increase in clearance ■ Food decreases bioavailability <30%	■ Drug tablets stable for at least 6 mo Cost of goods for API < $10K/kg	■ Some negotiation required with regulators after end-of-Phase II meeting. on design and size of pivotal efficacy and safety studies

Note: (AE) Adverse Event; (API) Active Pharmaceutical Ingredient; (AUC) Area Under the Curve; (CYP) Cytochrome; (SAE) Serious Adverse Event

Very disciplined decision-making processes are required to leverage the value of the decision gate approach. This begins by defining a clear set of questions at each decision gate that are agreed and understood by the decision makers. In the clinical stages of drug development, these questions and criteria are often presented in a Target Product Profile or TPP (see example, Table 3). The development program plan is assembled by determining: 1) which studies must be done and 2) their design that would provide information critical to answering key questions at each go/no go decision gate. Disciplined decision making involves the right people evaluating the information that is collected as the program is executed at the right time using an agreed upon process. Effective programs make decisions only when the required information is available, and once those decisions are made, rarely, if ever, is there a need to revisit them.

Managing productivity

Speed, quality and cost are the drivers of successful drug R&D process. There are a growing number of information technology tools supporting high-performance drug R&D, including data capture, project management, data management and others. The quality of program design can be a major factor in accelerated speed and quality by not wasting time and effort.

Outsourcing

The impact of outsourcing on pharmaceutical R&D is one of the major changes in the drug development process over the last decade. There is scarcely any part of the drug development process that has not been substantially outsourced, and an increasing number of companies are becoming 'virtual,' outsourcing every step of the process.

Contract research organizations (CROs) are legally defined in the U.S. by 21 CFR 312.3 as "a person that assumes, as an independent contractor with the sponsor, one or more of the obligations of a sponsor, e.g., design of a protocol, selection or monitoring

> The reasons for accelerated outsourcing in drug development are the same as the growth in outsourcing in other industry segments—enabling companies to expand their efforts without increasing their staff and facilities, focusing on areas of expertise and on developing the drug versus building infrastructure.

of investigations, evaluation of reports, and preparation of materials to be submitted to the Food and Drug Administration (FDA)."[7] This broad definition includes hundreds of organizations and professionals around the world supporting every aspect of sponsored drug research. The CRO market is estimated to be in excess of $15 billion with annual growth of 14-16%. Recent reports indicate that CRO-conducted clinical trials were completed 30% more quickly than those conducted in-house by the sponsor. Spending on outsourcing is growing consistently faster than the growth in development spending (Table 4), and headcount among major CROs between 2001 and 2004 grew 6% annually while sponsor (drug company) headcount remained level.

Table 4: Spending on Pharmaceutical Outsourcing vs Development (US$ Billion)

	2001	2002	2003	2004	3-yr Annualized Growth
Development Spending	$17.3	$30.1	$33.6	$37.7	11.2%
Contract Clinical Services	$3.7	$4.3	$4.9	$5.6	15.2%

The reasons for accelerated outsourcing in drug development are the same as the growth in outsourcing in other industry segments—enabling companies to expand their efforts without increasing their staff and facilities, focusing on areas of expertise and on developing the drug versus building infrastructure. More companies are conserving their cash to focus on the investment objective of bringing a new drug to an investment milestone vs. building fixed infrastructure costs. As more small–mid-tier pharma companies become clinical organizations, the high cost and low success ratio of human studies will create significant challenges for that sector, and lead them to adopt outsourcing and other clinical practices that big pharma is using to control costs and manage risk. Demand for CRO services is expected to grow by 16% annually for the next five years.

Will outsourcing growth continue in the contract research segment? Yes. Continued outsourcing growth will mean continued consolidation of the CRO industry. Growth in outsourcing will be driven by sustained growth in drug R&D, more complex clinical trials, increased pressures to manage the cost basis of a rapidly growing global biotechnology industry, the continued introduction of large numbers of potential drug candidates, expanded service offerings by CROs and globalization of the service offerings of more and more CROs.

The Future

Drivers that will shape Clinical Drug Development over the next 5-10 years include:

✦ Substantial health care and economic rewards for new medicine

✦ More sophisticated pharmaceutical science, management and information technology tools to increase development performance

✦ Globalization of markets and patient access. Post approval studies will limit patient access for clinical trials

✦ Integration of clinical care and clinical research to manage health care and drug development in the same process

✦ More complex clinical studies

✦ Outsourcing more relationship/alliance based than transaction based

References

1. I. Kola and J. Landis. *Can the Pharmaceutical Industry Reduce Attrition Rates?* Nature Reviews, Drug Discovery 3:711-715, 2004

2. *Parexel's Pharmaceutical R&D Statistical Sourcebook.*
    http://www.parexel.com/products/services/publications.asp

3. *Innovation Stagnation: Challenge and Opportunity on the Critical Path to New Medical Products.* US Food and Drug Administration. March 2004

4. *Monitoring Industrial Research: The 2007 EU Industrial R&D Investment Scoreboard.* European Commission Joint Research Center, October 2007

5. Hamm, Steve, *Business Week; Does R&D Deliver Results?* October 11, 2005

6. J. F. Pritchard, J. Jurima-Romet, M. Reimer, E. Mortimer, B. Rolfe, and M. Cayen, *Making Better Drugs: Decision Gaes in Non-Clinical Drug Development. Nature Reviews Drug Discovery* 2: 542-553, 2003.

7. *Code of Federal Regulations*, Title 21, Volume 5. 21 CFR 312.3

8. *Tufts Center for the Study of Drug Development,* Outlook 2007

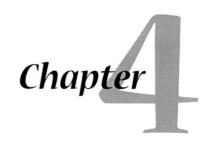

Chapter 4

Clinical trial process – project management

Ms. Jan Robinson, PharmaKodex Ltd.

> Rapid decision-making and the
> ability to modify the plans and
> invoke new strategies to implement
> the required changes are essential.

Background

The ultimate goal for pharmaceutical and biotechnology companies is to gain approval to market their drug. Once the ink is dry on a company's clinical trials strategy document, someone has to plan and deliver the trials that will provide the data for filings to regulatory bodies worldwide. Project management involves planning, conducting and reporting these trials; all of which are critical to the company's success. The clinical trial process is governed by a plethora of complex regulations and guidelines. Moreover, understanding the nuances of conducting trials in individual countries is an important factor. Although these cross-border requirements are generally similar, in practice, understanding the legal requirements and following the laws in individual countries is not always harmonious.

> **The ultimate goal for pharmaceutical and biotechnology companies is to gain approval to market their drug.**

What is a project manager

The role of project managers in the pharmaceutical industry depends on the responsibility their company requires of them within the clinical trial process. Project managers may be responsible for delivering a relatively small part of a single trial or a whole suite of trials. They may be working for the sponsor pharmaceutical or biotechnology company or for one of the service provider contract research organizations (CROs) responsible for executing a clinical trial. As such, Project Managers often exist in multiple tiers across projects, each responsible for a set of individual deliverables. Some examples include a Project Manager:

✦ within the sponsor pharmaceutical/biotechnology company responsible for defining the strategy and delivering the whole program of trials

✦ responsible for delivering one or more of the trials either within the pharmaceutical company or working in a service provider CRO

✦ at a Phase I unit responsible for co-ordinating all the activities at the unit and interfacing with a Project Manager in the sponsor pharmaceutical company or CRO

✦ at a Site Management Organization (SMO) responsible for ensuring recruitment and management of patients at that particular site or at multiple sites and the delivery of the data to the sponsor or other CRO

✦ responsible for ensuring that conduct of the trial at all the individual sites is being monitored by suitable qualified trial monitors, ensuring standardization across sites and countries and compliance with all the legal requirements and the trial protocol

✦ in the data management department responsible for management of the tools to capture the data, clean, store, analyse and report them

✦ responsible for co-ordinating the delivery of blood kits to all the sites, co-ordinating return by courier, processing, analysis and reporting of the results to a central database.

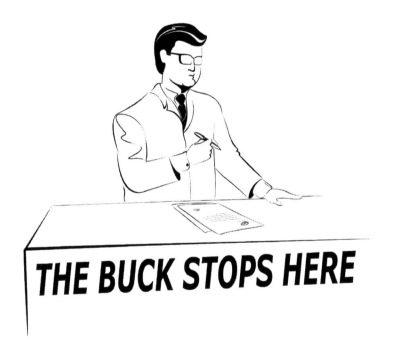

Confusingly, the title Project Manager is widely misused in the industry and hence you will find people with titles such as Clinical Trial Manager, Program Manager, Project Director, Project Co-ordinator, Medical Program Co-ordinators, Project Leaders. How much they perform true project management as compared to just executing clinical trial tasks depends on their role. A Project Leader, for example, may be looking at the big picture and linking sponsor, project team and senior management. A Project Manager may be responsible for the day-to-day deliverables of the trial.

Whatever the case, there are two capability sets required for an effective Project Manager within the pharmaceutical industry:

1. an ability to use generic skills of project management and

2. a thorough understanding and experience of those parts of the clinical trial process for which they are responsible.

The breadth of knowledge required with regard to the clinical trial process will depend on the definition of the "project" for the individual within the context of the clinical trials program. The basic precepts for project management apply in the pharmaceutical industry in just the same way as any other industry and fall into the following categories:

◆ Defining the scope and planning
◆ Assessing the feasibility
◆ Assessing and monitoring resource requirements and time and cost
◆ Organizing and leading the team(s) responsible for delivery of the project
◆ Risk Management
◆ Monitoring and controlling progress and resolving conflict
◆ Closing out at conclusion

Defining scope and planning

Clinical development plan

Many of the critical decisions and tasks that lead to a successful pharmaceutical project are front-loaded and the study set up period is one of intense activity. Most pharmaceutical companies start with a clinical development plan. This is a document that describes all the activities pertaining to the development of a product and may include regulatory and commercial strategies, various project plans for the trials, the budget, forecasting of resource and the operational feasibility.

The definition of the project scope usually happens within the pharmaceutical company, although for some very small start-up companies the task may be assigned to a consultancy or CRO, or developed collaboratively. Significant input is required from numerous departments, often across multiple organizations. The scope of the project is defined at a top level and considers the whole suite of studies. The key activities and timelines are identified and documented. A detailed breakdown is then developed considering the overall objectives and the discrete tasks that will have to be accomplished. Key milestones are decided. These milestones represent points at which something critical to the project schedule will have been achieved that gates the progression of the study. These milestones may include such things as obtaining regulatory and ethics approvals to allow the study to commence, enrolling the first patient (or for Phase I healthy volunteer) to the study, the last patient completing the study, the date of locking of the clinical database or the date when the final clinical study report is to be signed off and all the sites and files are closed.

Much emphasis is given to the critical path through the trial because in terms of management this is what determines the total duration of the trial and that is the key to commercial success.

> **Many of the critical decisions and tasks that lead to a successful pharmaceutical project are front-loaded and the study set-up period is one of intense activity.**

So in short, the project manager, usually with the help of a multi-functional supporting team, defines the scope, the objectives, the individual goals and the expected outcomes of a project. He or she also identifies all the resources needed, at what cost and within what timeframe. Thereafter, the Project Manager must ensure that the plan is implemented, manage the expectations of all the stakeholders in the project, monitor and track progress and 'pull a rabbit out of the hat' when things go wrong, which they frequently do!

Quality standards

The quality standards to be adopted are also defined during planning. They are essential to ensure the integrity of the data and the safety of the participant patients or healthy volunteers. If activities are to be outsourced there will be discussion regarding whose standard operating procedures will be applied and what training is needed to ensure standardization across multiple sites and how to maintain a high level of quality. Standardization and training are critical particularly for large Phase III pivotal trials conducted in multiple countries. The last thing the pharmaceutical company wants is data that show that when the same treatment is given to the same type of patients in the same way, it results in a different outcome in a different country. Many a Phase III program has been sunk because of small differences in the way the protocol for the trial was actually applied in a particular country. This can be due to subtle differences in medical practice that can impact the data and provide a result different from the one expected.

Cost planning

A set of costs is built for the trial together with a pro forma spends and a process for monitoring and tracking that spend. This may be simple task for a Phase I study but can be a gargantuan challenge for larger studies with hundreds of sites spread across the globe.

> Many a Phase III program has been sunk because of small differences in the way the protocol for the trial was actually applied in a particular country.

Planning tools

In order to meet the challenges of planning and execution, project management needs tools to assist them. Decisions are made as to what types of information management systems are going to be used, exactly what information is to be stored, where and how it will be stored, how it is to be tracked and to whom it needs to be made available during the study. All the stakeholders are interested in the study and the recipients may be anyone from senior management, marketing or corporate communications as well as the trial team members themselves. At its simplest, a Phase I study may only require Excel spreadsheets, Gantt charts and tables. The tools available to project management is evolving and large pharmaceutical companies have their own clinical trial management systems for managing sites, fee/grant payment processes, tracking recruitment, storing regulatory documentation, study monitoring tracking, project team resourcing and budgeting and status and project reports. The use of Web portals to permit real time access to information to authorized users is now common.

Trial feasibility assessment

Assessing the feasibility of a trial is important for effective project management. All plans are based on assumptions and these assumptions can, to some extent, be tested before the actual trial begins. Project management needs to know whether the trial can be done practically and successfully. Questions that need answering may include:

+ Does the defined population actually exist?
+ Are the countries being considered the most likely to be able provide investigators to recruit efficiently and perform effectively?
+ Is the timeline realistic?
+ What service providers are the best ones to use?
+ What data capture technologies are the most appropriate?

At its simplest, feasibility involves supplying experienced trial sites with a protocol outline and asking them whether they think the execution would be realistic and within what timeframe they believe patients or volunteers could be recruited. Sometimes complete end-to-end pilot feasibility studies are conducted to test assumptions before embarking on expensive and risk-laden trials.

> **A detailed breakdown of the plan including a tasks network and a skills matrix is often developed to assist with resource planning.**

Assessing resource requirements

A detailed breakdown of the plan including a tasks network and a skills matrix is often developed to assist with resource planning. There has to be a decision as to where the staff will be sourced, which aspects of the trial will be done in-house and what will be outsourced to CROs. Core competencies will be identified particularly in relation to the critical path of the trial. If outsourcing is part of the plan then an identification, selection and qualification process for contractors has to be decided. A resource management plan may be produced to forecast possible delays, provide contingency and allow for the anticipated turnover of staff during the trial. The allocation of responsibilities is broken down and assigned to ensure that the legal and regulatory requirements can be met and all the deliverables achieved.

Organizing and leading the team

Once the project plan defining the deliverables and milestones is prepared the Project Manager has to organize, lead and control the execution of the trial to ensure that all the goals are achieved on time and on budget. One can equate this to the conductor of an orchestra who, though they do not have to play a single instrument themselves, must annotate the music in detail, ensure everyone is equipped to play their part, make sure they are all in tune before the opening bars and conduct them so that they all come in and out at the right moment. If the conductor can hold it all together, the ultimate goal, a perfect performance, is the likely outcome.

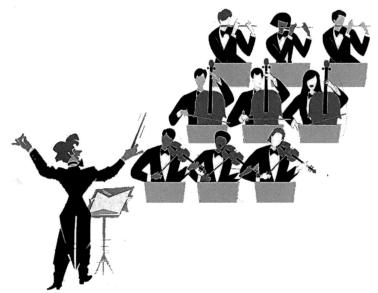

Leading the team is sometimes likened to a conductor leading the orchestra.

The Project Manager needs their team, or more often multiple teams, all contributing different deliverables as part of the master project plan. The teams may be internal at the Sponsor Company or external involving CRO participation if responsibilities are outsourced. So, a key competency for a good Project Manager is the ability to build and motivate a team and manage interactions across multiple levels of the organizations and across multiple disciplines both internally and externally. Projects fail more often due to human issues than anything else and good communication, strong teamwork, negotiation, problem solving and conflict resolution are essential. The project team has to monitor the duration of tasks and the resources and keep the channels of communication constantly flowing.

The set-up phase of a trial is a period of intense activity and it is during this phase that the team will generate most of the key documents required for trial conduct. It is not within the scope of this chapter to discuss all the documentation required but the investigator's brochure, protocol and case record form are critical documents worth understanding.

Investigator's brochure

The investigator's brochure is a compilation of both the non-clinical and clinical data known about the drug that is relevant to the proposed trial in human subjects. It will describe animal results predicting human toxicity and any preclinical animal studies including pharmacology, pharmacokinetics, mutagenicity, reproductive toxicology and carcinogenicity potential. In short, it attempts to summarize all the data known about the product under test and assists the investigator, ethical and regulatory bodies in deciding that it is ethically and scientifically reasonable to conduct the trial and that there is an adequate safety margin for the trial to proceed. Given the contents, it is easy to see that the investigator's brochure requires input from a variety of functions and the generation of the document usually occurs within the pharmaceutical company and is often co-ordinated by a physician or project manager. If the drug in question already has a history of safe use, information in the investigator's brochure may reference data already in the public domain.

Protocol

The 'master plan' for the study is the protocol. This document is typically 50-100 pages long. It describes the hypothesis and purpose of the trial, the exact nature of the population who will receive the test products, the medical condition they must be suffering from, the criteria participants have to fulfil to be eligible, the organization of the trial, the tests and procedures to be conducted and the means of analyzing and reporting. The protocol will have team input from a variety of sources including, for example:

> The 'master plan' for the study is the protocol.

+ Physicians involved in the study

✦ Biostatisticians who justify the trial size and specify the data collection and analysis requirements

✦ Regulatory affairs staff that check country specific regulatory requirements and the clinical trial drug supply department.

The design of the protocol will differ depending on the phase of the study and the indication for the drug (the specific medical condition that the drug is intended to treat). The protocol will define whether the study is 'open' which means that everyone knows what treatment each patient is receiving or blinded in some way which means that some parties will not know what the patient is receiving. Sometimes a study is referred to as double blind to prevent any bias that could influence the conduct, collection and analysis of the data. Usually another, alternative treatment is incorporated to provide a comparison. This may be a placebo (something that looks like the drug under test but has no active ingredient in it) or there may be another comparator such a drug already on the market.

To prevent bias, treatments need to be allocated randomly and the methods used to achieve this can be simple or very complex depending on the trial size and complexity. Interactive web or voice response systems are now common where, once a participant is confirmed as eligible, the treatment is assigned following a phone or fax call or web interaction from the investigational site to a central hub where randomization is controlled. The protocol may dictate the design of the study as parallel where different groups of participants get different treatment in parallel or a cross over design where the same subject may get one treatment after another with a period in between to allow the effects of the previous treatment to wear off. The protocol would state the conditions for escalation from one dose to another if that was appropriate. The sample size has to be justified in the protocol so that the number of subjects included is likely to give a clear indication that the original hypothesis for the trial can be proved and has to take into account the effects of multiple centers and treatments and other factors influencing the likely variability of the data.

Case record form

Once the protocol is available, the case report form or case record form (CRF) is designed. The CRF can be a printed, optical or electronic document and is designed to capture all the data required by the protocol for a particular patient in an unambiguous way. The data within the CRF confirm that the patient fulfils the eligibility criteria, contains all the information regarding medical diagnosis, any baseline (pre treatment) assessments, the treatment details and the results of all the tests that the protocol states must be performed for each participant in order to assess the response to the treatment. Confusingly, the term CRF can sometimes refer to either just one page or all the data for an individual subject.

Other documents

The investigator's brochure and protocol are just two of the documents that must be prepared during the set up phase in order to obtain the necessary ethical and regulatory approvals for the study to proceed in the chosen countries. International guidelines require that all trials be reviewed and approved before exposing patients (or volunteers) to the hazards of trial participation. Review of the trial is always conducted by an ethics committee, called an Institutional Review Board (IRB) in the USA or Ethics Committee in Europe, to ensure the rights and safety of participants in clinical trials. Ethical review may result in the granting of approval but just as frequently in requests to change the trial procedure in some way or sometimes even deny approval in the country question. From a project management perspective delays due to ethics review are common, difficult to predict and can cause havoc with the predicted timelines for a trial.

> From a project management perspective delays due to ethics review are common, difficult to predict and can cause havoc with the predicted timelines for a trial.

Site selection

Another important activity during study set up is the identification of the trial sites and the investigators who will participate. The Principal Investigator is the medically qualified person at the trial site responsible for the conduct of the study. He or she is often assisted by multiple sub- or co-investigators. Identification of properly trained, qualified, and experienced investigators to perform the trial is vital to its outcome. During the set up period qualification of sites and staff will confirm that the investigator has the necessary facilities to do the trial procedures, fully understands how the drug is to be used and what the safety profile is, including any known side effects that may occur.

The key stakeholders for a study will usually attend a start up meeting that typically includes a training element. The project plan will be communicated; the milestones, recruitment expectations, timelines, the roles and responsibilities within the trial process, the quality standards, monitoring guidelines, management of drug treatments, assessments, safety procedures and more will be covered. There will be written plans for control of documentation and for communication flow. The nature of the communication, format, type, method, and frequency will all be discussed, often in exquisite detail. For large studies multiple teams will exist in different countries all feeding into a core team functioning as the central command unit usually within the pharmaceutical company or the CRO.

Risk management

Conducting clinical trials is not always a straightforward process and good planning alone does not always assure you will hit the finishing line, at the right time, every time. The chances of a clinical trial finishing on time are much the same as winning the Kentucky Derby. Approximately 80% of trials are delayed when compared with the original expectation. The reason is that the process is littered with risk from start to finish. One of the major challenges for project management is to identify the important risks that will have the

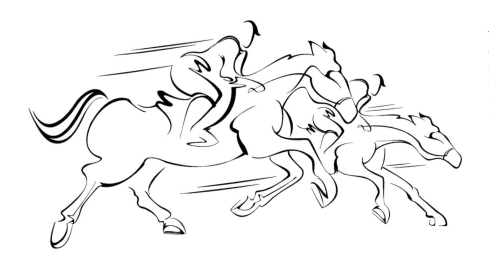

The chances of a clinical trial finishing on time are much the same as winning the Kentucky Derby.
Illustration by Wadi Talhami, NY

greatest impact on the objectives and try and build in contingency from the planning stage. Most companies conduct some kind of risk management process to assess the probabilities and consequences of the undesirable happening.

The risk is quantified based on the project plan and a process is established to track and review the risks as the study progresses. There are plenty of classic examples of inherent risk in any clinical trial. For example risks at study start may include:

+ Delays in the regulatory bodies granting permission to start the trial until further information is provided.
+ Ethical committees or Institutional Review Boards may delay the trial until their questions receive appropriate answers.
+ Recruitment of volunteers or patients is frequently much slower than was anticipated and is often quoted as the primary one reason for late completion of trials. This can be due to a host of reasons such as a time slippage invoking a clash with other studies recruiting similar patients, over optimism by investigators or new treatments being unexpectedly available which make participation in the study less attractive.

Wise project management builds in contingency in terms of additional budget and /or time at the planning stage and defines at what point the contingency will be used.

Progress control and resolving conflict

We have described how project management is responsible for initiating systems to assess progress and performance against the common goals that have been agreed to by the pharmaceutical company and their CRO. This constant tracking of progress is essential to initiate 'rescue' measures if things do not proceed as planned. Problem-shooting must be available in the arsenal of any good Project Manager in order to deal with the inevitable variance. Rapid decision-making and the ability to modify the plans and invoke new strategies to implement the required changes are essential. The Project Manager also has to resolve conflicts arising between any of the stakeholders. The pressure to drive down costs has led to fewer face-to-face meetings, and the scope for conflict is therefore enhanced particularly when cultural differences are taken into account. Managing multinational teams

> **The Project Manager also has to resolve conflicts arising between any of the stakeholders.**

is difficult and conflict emerges logarithmically with more remote communication. As virtual meetings become more common the chances of conflict arising are increased not decreased unless there is effective management.

Closing Out

At the end of the study the most important deliverable is the *integrated clinical study report*, which encompasses the complete scientific record of the trial. The report becomes part of any submission for marketing authorization worldwide and is written in accordance with guidelines.

While the report is being prepared, reviewed and approved all the project documentation has to be transferred to the sponsor and the sites closed down. Traditionally much of the clinical trial data was paper based but the move toward electronic data capture is accelerating. Clinical trials are paper mountains and the trial master file for even a small study is frequently 50-100 beer-crate sized boxes. A single large study can be hundreds of boxes. Often the sponsor company will conduct a review and learning session to examine the scars inflicted by the study, document the achievements and all the knowledge that has been gained in order to apply it to future trials. The data from the trials are then combined into integrated reports summarizing all the safety and efficacy data on the product in an attempt to secure permission from regulatory bodies to market the drug. Project management continues after the drug has obtained marketing approval in one country to expand to territories where the drug can be marketed. In addition, further trials are also developed and conducted to expand the indications and patient populations in which it can be used.

The costs of pharmaceutical development are accelerating at an alarming rate and the industry is looking to project management to provide savings in terms of time and cost. Project planning is becoming more flexible and will have to be more creative to provide the solutions necessary to deliver enhanced performance. Better risk management and planning for uncertainty will be essential facets in achieving this goal.

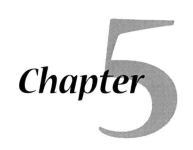

Chapter 5

Primer on Ethics in Clinical Research

Felix A. Khin-Maung-Gyi, PharmD, MBA, CIP, RAC

Chief Executive Officer/Founder Chesapeake Research Review, Inc. Columbia, Maryland, USA

> "Those who cannot remember
> the past are condemned
> to repeat it."
> — *George Santayana*
> *Life of Reason, Reason in Common Sense,*
> Scribner's, 1905, p. 284

Background

Professionals who are fortunate enough to conduct research involving human research participants have a great opportunity to benefit society and add to the generalized knowledge that is the basis for scientific breakthroughs. Yet, with this opportunity comes a humbling responsibility. All of us should be continually mindful of the fact that what we do is feasible only because individual human beings have given us permission to expose them to risks. These risks, no matter how big or small, are inherent to research. Participants who agree to enroll in a study do so because they want to help others and to promote science. However, they also do it because they trust that researchers will honor their personal sacrifice and use it solely for the common good. As research professionals, we make a personal promise to do so when we obtain a person's informed consent at the time of enrollment into the study.

> **All of us should be continually mindful of the fact that what we do is feasible only because individual human beings have given us permission to expose them to risks.**

In the United States, and other countries that have a governmental structure to enact legislation and subsequent regulation, there are regulations that specifically assure the protection of the rights and welfare of those participating in clinical research. In the United States, these include separate regulations governing research that is funded by the federal government and by private sponsors conducting research involving products regulated by the US Food and Drug Administration (FDA).[1,2] Both were published in the Federal Register and promulgated in 1981. In an effort to harmonize regulations around the world, the International Conference on Harmonisation (ICH) issued guidelines for the appropriate protections of research participants.[3] Collectively, these regulations and guidelines are referred to as "Good Clinical Practice (GCP)."

Protection of research subjects has not always been regulated, however. The current regulations are based on ethical principles and codes that have been established and adopted by the research community over the course of the last century.[4,5,6] Many of these standards were set after a series of tragedies was directly linked to the conduct of either biomedical or social science/behavioral research and most have been in existence for only a relatively short period considering the long history of clinical research.

In the U.S., the current human subject protections regulations are based, in large measure, on the Belmont Report issued in 1979[7]. This report was the product of the National Commission for the Protection of Human Subjects of Biomedical and Behavioral Research that was created by the U.S. Congress when it passed the National Research Act on July 12, 1974. Congress established the Commission to address the scandal created by the now infamous "Tuskegee syphilis study" that was sponsored and conducted by the U.S. Public Health Service.[8,9]

The Belmont Report outlines three ethical principles that must be considered in the conduct of research: respect for persons, beneficence and justice. In application, these three principles respectively, translate to:

1. obtaining and documenting informed consent;

2. adequately assessing the risk benefit of the proposed research; and

3. selecting subjects appropriately so that the population bearing the risk of participation in the study is the same population that will benefit from the information gathered in the trial.

The Belmont Report suggests that the protection of study subjects is a shared responsibility that involves the investigator and other study staff. In practice, the Institutional Review Board (IRB) or Ethics Committee (EC) remains the primary gatekeeper as defined by the regulations and guided by the application of ethical principles.

Principles and codes for ethical conduct of clinical research have existed since the early 1900's[10,11] but the actual establishment and application of regulations that govern human research protections did not occur until the early 1980s. The regulations regarding the protection of human research participants that have been enacted by federal officials in the U.S. are cited as standard and are the basis for regulations promulgated in other countries that conduct clinical research as well as international standards. For this reason, it is worthwhile to examine the history that preceded the Belmont Report and led to its enactment.

> **In practice, the Institutional Review Board (IRB) or Ethics Committee (EC) remains the primary gatekeeper as defined by the regulations and guided by the application of ethical principles.**

On the Road to Belmont: A Brief Historical Perspective

The history of "applied ethics in research" can have many starting points but because informed consent is most widely viewed by the research community as the cornerstone of the ethical conduct of research, we begin this rich history with the work of one of the best-known and respected researchers who first used informed consent – Dr. Walter Reed. There are a number of other historical treatises on the subject of applied ethics in research.[12,13,14,15,1617]

Dr. Reed used one of the first known informed consent documents when he enrolled participants, including medical personnel, in his study that purposely exposed them to the disease. Dr. Reed led the U.S. Army's Yellow Fever Commission that was attempting to decrease the high mortality from the disease that had become widespread in Cuba during the Spanish-American War and was threatening the ability to build the Panama Canal. Participants were given a one-page informed consent document in either English or Spanish that briefly outlined the risks of participation in Dr. Reed's study as well as the monetary compensation that each participant would receive.

> Dr. Reed used one of the first known informed consent documents when he enrolled participants, including medical personnel, in his study that purposely exposed them to the disease.

The notion of informed consent was not always applied in the way we expect it will be today. In 1932, another U.S. governmental agency, the U.S. Public Health Service (USPHS), began a clinical trial that lasted over 40 years and is known not for its medical advancement but rather as an example of coercion, deception and an egregious breech of professional conduct. The USPHS Study of the Natural Sequela of Tertiary Syphilis in Elderly and Poorly Educated African American Males (the official name of the study) in rural Macon County, Alabama is known today as the Tuskegee syphilis study.

Subjects were 400 African American sharecroppers with latent syphilis and 200 African American men who did not have the disease when they enrolled and who served as a control group for the trial. The participants were promised treatment for their disease but received none even though penicillin was discovered eight years after the study began. The USPHS researchers purposely told physicians in neighboring Alabama counties not to treat the men with late-stage syphilis and promised the study participants that the government would pay for their burial expenses if they agreed to enroll in the trial.

The USPHS study was stopped in 1972 when a Peter Buxtun, a psychiatric social worker for the USPHS in San Francisco, exposed the details to an Associated Press reporter and it was published in the *Washington Star* among other newspapers.

Although the exact number of deaths is not known, one author who conducted a case study of the USPHS study estimates that as many as 100 men died "as a direct result of complications caused by syphilis," and additional deaths can be traced to complications such as coronary heart disease.[8] The study at Tuskegee is also important to understand because the distrust for research among African Americans that it created continues to a lesser degree even today. "The Tuskegee Study is America's metaphor for racism in medical research," said one historian.[9]

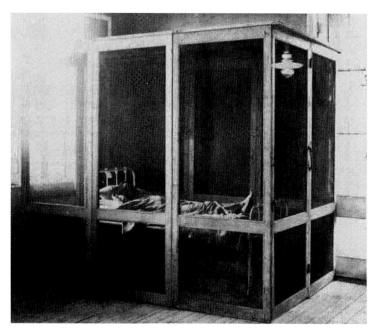

1905 Yellow Fever Quarantine Station. Credit: Panama Canal History Museum.

Unethical conduct in the name of clinical research was not confined to the U.S alone. One of the most flagrant abuses of human subjects was the enrollment of prisoners in concentration camps in Nazi Germany during World War II. Nazi doctors conducted these experiments on non-German nationals, including Jews and "asocial" persons. After the war ended, the Nuremberg Trials exposed these abuses and, subsequently, the Nuremberg Code was issued in 1947. It lists 10 basic principles of ethical research including the first principle that is now considered the key element of informed consent.

The Nuremberg Trials surfaced the conduct of these trials that included the injection of prisoners with gasoline and live viruses, the exposing of people to extremely cold temperatures and pressure (altitude), the infliction of wounds to test various treatments and the forced-ingestion of poisons.

Although it was initially not widely accepted in the international medical community, the Nuremberg Code established a benchmark that has been repeated throughout other sentinel documents and regulations on human research protections. The first tenet of the Code formalizes a standard for informed and voluntary consent of the research participant. (See shaded Box on this page).

The 20th century includes other examples of unethical conduct in trials in the U.S. as well as other events that triggered the establishment of new ethical principles and government guidance and regulation. A brief history in addition to the Tuskegee study, Belmont Report and the Nuremberg Code includes the following[13,14,16,17]:

The first tenet of the Nuremberg Code

The voluntary consent of the human subject is absolutely essential. This means that the person involved should have legal capacity to give consent; should be so situated as to be able to exercise free power of choice, without the intervention of any element of force, fraud, deceit, duress, over-reaching, or other ulterior form of constraints or coercion; and should have sufficient knowledge and comprehension of the elements of the subject matter involved as to enable him to make an understanding and enlightened decision. This latter element requires that before the acceptance of an affirmative decision by the experimental subject there should be make know to him the nature, duration, and purpose of the inconveniences and hazards reasonable to be expected; and the effects upon h is health or person which may possibly come from his participation in the experiment.

The duty and responsibility for ascertaining the quality of the consent rests upon each individual who initiates, directs or engages in the experiment. It is a personal duty and responsibility which may not be delegated to another with impunity.

✦ 1953/4 – The Wichita Jury Study was led by researchers at the University of Chicago and involved the unethical act of recording jury deliberations without their knowledge or consent. The judge and lawyers in the trial approved of the practice that was later prohibited by Congress.

✦ 1963 – Sloan Kettering/Jewish Chronic Disease Hospital researchers in Brooklyn, NY, injected live cancer cells into elderly and debilitated patients without their consent.

✦ Early 1960's – Willowbrook State School, Willowbrook, NY researchers injected hepatitis virus into pediatric patients with mental retardation. The physician investigators did obtain the informed consent of the parents of these children but they later said they were told that their child was given a vaccine. Parents also said that they were forced to agree to the injection as a condition of the child's acceptance into the care of the institution.

✦ 1964- Dr. Stanley Milgram's social psychology research at Yale University. The intent of the study was to determine the willingness of a person to obey an order and the driving factors behind disobedience and obedience to authority. Subjects were brought into a laboratory and subsequently asked questions. If they gave the wrong answer they received what they thought was an electric shock. The "shocks" increased with each incorrect answer. Although the subjects were debriefed and informed that they did not actually receive shocks, the study was criticized for its deception. The research community addressed concerns about this type of trial by clarifying when a waiver of informed consent is appropriate.

Note: The experiment's true ("naive") subjects were brought into a laboratory and each instructed to ask questions of a purported experimental subject ("learner") who was actually an accomplice of the investigator.

Government regulations

Federal regulations in the U.S. are derived from the Belmont Report and from a 1962 amendment to law called the Kefauver-Harris Amendments to the Federal Food, Drug and Cosmetic Act. (See Chapter on the History of the FDA.) The amendments require that informed consent be obtained from any participant in a study of experimental drugs that is conducted under government (Food and Drug Administration [FDA]) oversight.

Federal regulations governing research conduct that is FDA regulated are published in Title 21 of the Code of Federal Regulations. These regulations were established in 1981 and cover research trials that are sponsored by non-government entities such as drug, medical device and biologics manufacturers. The FDA regulations are listed in two separate parts: 21 CFR 50 outlines requirements for the protection of human subjects including that for informed consent. 21 CFR 56 outlines requirements for clinical trials and for the role of IRBs.

Federal regulations governing research conduct that is funded by the federal government, including the National Institutes of Health, the Department of Defense, Department of Energy and other federal agencies, are published in Title 45 of the Code of Federal Regulations, Part 46. They were published in 1981 as well and are divided into Subparts A-D. Subpart A includes basic requirements for human subject protection. Subpart B outlines special protections pertaining to research development, and related activities involving fetuses, pregnant women, and human in vitro fertilization. Subpart C outlines additional protections pertaining to biomedical and behavioral research involving prisoners as subjects. Subpart D provides additional protections for children involved as subjects in research.

> **Federal regulations governing research conduct that is FDA regulated are published in Title 21 of the Code of Federal Regulations.**

Federal regulations including 45 CFR 46, 21 CFR 50 and 21 CFR 56 have all been amended and are continually under review and analysis by government officials including the U.S. Department of Health and Human Services (DHHS, http://www.hhs.gov/), FDA (http://www.fda.gov), the Office of Human Research Protections (OPHRP, http://www.hhs.gov/ohrp/) and the Secretary's Advisory Committee for Human Research Protections (SACHRP, http://www.hhs.gov/ohrp/sachrp/

index.html), a federal advisory panel that offers recommendations to the Secretary of DHHS.

In 1964, the World Medical Assembly that was meeting in Helsinki, Finland, issued what is called the Helsinki Declaration. It focuses on the relationship between the physician as investigator and the study participant. It has been revised several times since its initial publication – most recently in October 2000 with additional clarifications in 2004 (http://www.wma.net/e/policy/b3.htm).

> **In 1964, the World Medical Assembly that was meeting in Helsinki, Finland, issued what is called the Helsinki Declaration.**

In 1996, International Committee on Harmonisation (ICH) issued a publication entitled, "Guideline for Good Clinical Practice." The document includes informed consent recommendations. Its goal is to harmonize clinical research regulations in the U.S, Europe and Japan (http://www.ich.org/cache/compo/276-254-1.html).

Training and education

Not every ethical lapse in clinical research today is as blatant a violation of human subject protection as the startling examples outlined here that shape our collective thinking. Today's questions that must be answered by the entire research team, including the sponsor, investigator research staff, IRB and the regulatory agencies are these:

◆ Would we necessarily recognize unethical behavior when we see it?

◆ Would we likely recognize unethical behavior *and* a lot of the gray area in between?

◆ Are there factors that potentially can, or unwittingly do, lead clinical research professionals astray as they conduct clinical research activities with every intention of meaning to do well by the research participant?

Certainly one factor, in particular, is a lack of education and training. In 2000, the National Institutes of Health implemented a policy that requires education on human subject protection for all investigators and 'key personnel' that have responsibilities for the design and conduct of a clinical trial. The NIH does not mandate a specific training program but it does require the investigator to document in annual progress reports and in all cover letters that research staff has met these requirements.

But training alone is not sufficient to address the range of decision making encountered in the clinical research enterprise. By its nature, ethical behavior is not defined in algorithmic simple "do's" and "don'ts". Similarly, professionals trained in medicine, nursing, and other clinical and/or administrative fields do not automatically have the expertise to understand the complex nature of clinical research especially in relation to the practice of clinical medcine.

There are many potential conflicts of interests in the clinical setting, a number of which stem from an inherent conflict of roles. Physician investigators, in particular, have a conflicting role between being a caregiver and a researcher. The primary motivation of the clinician caregiver is the health and medical treatment of the patient; the primary motivation of the clinician researcher is the advancement of science and collection of data. The Belmont Report helps us to differentiate between clinical research and clinical medicine. (See shaded Box on this page).

The Belmont Report [5]

"For the most part, the term "practice" refers to interventions that are designed solely to enhance the well-being of an individual patient or client and that have a reasonable expectation of success. The purpose of medical or behavioral practice is to provide diagnosis, preventive treatment or therapy to particular individuals. By contrast, the term "research' designates an activity designed to test an hypothesis, permit conclusions to be drawn, and thereby to develop or contribute to generalizable knowledge (expressed, for example, in theories, principles, and statements of relationships). Research is usually described in a formal protocol that sets forth an objective and a set of procedures designed to reach that objective."

Those achieving professional certification demonstrate that they have a basic understanding of core principles, if not competencies, relating to research regulations and ethical principles. However, investigators, clinical research coordinators, clinical research associates, data monitors, IRB members, and other research staff can and do make mistakes because of a lack of understanding, or experience, in interpreting regulations or applying ethical principles. The former head of the Office of Protection from Research Risks (OPRR, now OHRP), Gary Ellis, PhD, wrote in 1999, "There is no upper limit to the amount of information about the nuances of protecting the rights and welfare of research subjects. There is always more to learn, for example, about communicating risk to protect subjects in the consent process, about crafting language understandable to the subject, or about protecting the privacy of subjects and the confidentiality of personally identifiable information."[18]

Ethics, morals and professional behavior

In order for research professionals to conduct research in an ethical manner, they are required to be more than familiar with the federal regulations regarding human subject protection. Ezekiel Emmanuel, MD, PhD, Chair, Department of Clinical Bioethics at the National Institutes of Health, and his colleagues have delineated what they refer to as basic elements required to conduct ethical clinical research.[19]

Emanuel and his colleagues emphasize that although informed consent is a cornerstone of ethical research obtaining consent from a participant does not, in and of itself, mean that the entire research study is ethical. Other ethical concerns may include appropriate and adequate study design, fair subject selection, appropriate risk benefit ratios, the value of research to the individual and to society as a whole.

They recommend seven requirements for the ethical conduct of research. They are as follows:

1. **Value** – Well-trained clinical professionals who want to do clinical research should ask a fundamental question: "Does the research hypothesis/question enhance health or scientific/clinical knowledge?" It is unethical to expose someone to risk in a study if there is no value. The data from a study based on an investigator's hypothesis, for example, is unlikely to provide generalizable knowledge as required by federal regulations governing research. Likewise, a study may lead to further scientific inquiry but have no practical application in daily medical practice. Emanuel contends that value must exist as an ethical requirement because the willingness of research subjects to participate should not be exploited and there are finite funding sources for research that should be used with discretion.

2. **Scientific validity** – Even a study with the greatest potential for scientific discovery – a cure for cancer – may be ethically questionable if the study design does not assure scientific validity. The study design must be methodologically rigorous and assure that the study results in "clean" data and information that is "generalizable". In addition to the investigator of the study, the knowledge and expertise of other professionals is essential to this requirement. For example, the Clinical Research Associate (CRA) must be trained and follow good clinical practice. The CRA must apply clinical logic in monitoring the integrity of the data that is collected at the research site and should know basic scientific and clinical principles such as pharmacokinetic and pharmacodynamic concepts, dosing intervals, classes of drugs, uses of drugs and possible drug interactions. The IRB membership must include someone with training and expertise in the study area. In order for the IRB to discharge its responsibilities under federal law, the members must be trained to understand all aspects of the research program. For example, the scientific validity of a pediatric oncology protocol may not be adequately determined by a group that does not include a pediatric oncologist or if the IRB has not been trained/sensitized to clinical or ethical issues in this specialized area. If IRB members do not have the knowledge and expertise to determine the scientific validity of a protocol they must seek the advice of an outside consultant with these credentials and ability.

3. **Fair subject selection** – "Justice", according to the Belmont Report, speaks to the notion of exposing harms of research to the population who would ultimately benefit. In ethical terms this is "distributive justice." Emanuel argues that groups or individuals should never be targeted for study participation, nor should they be excluded because their participation may present logistical problems for the study staff. Groups or individuals who will not benefit from the research study should not bear the burden of participation rather than others who do stand to benefit. Science and risk/benefit analyses should be used to determine who should be included or not included in a particular study. It is also not ethical to enroll subjects based on factors that have no relevance to the study (e.g. enrolling

someone who has no health insurance so that s/he can obtain health care). Emanuel suggests that investigators ask several questions to determine whether a potential subject should be enrolled – Is the potential participant already enrolled in another trial? Will this second trial participation conflict with the first study participation? Is there any increased risk to subjects enrolled in more than one trial without a wash-out period? Can the possible participant benefit if s/he does not have access to follow-up medical care?

4. **Favorable risk-benefit ratio** – If there is no benefit in the study and/or if the risks are egregious, it may be unethical, says Emanuel, to enroll subjects. Risk and benefits must be outlined in the protocol and the design must minimize these risks as much as possible. A small possible benefit cannot outweigh a serious clinical risk.

5. **Independent review** – Review, approval and oversight by independent review (e.g. an IRB or EC) should take place only after the first four of these requirements are met. Investigators, research coordinators, monitors, sponsors, IRBs all face conflicts at various stages of a study that may hinder their independence. Education and appropriate allocation of resources to provide ongoing training and education of IRB staff greatly contribute to assuring this independence.

> Overall, Emanuel and his fellow ethicists conclude that these seven requirements are universal in nature and, thus, pertain to all research studies.

6. **Informed consent** – In order for consent to be informed, Emanuel says the potential participant must understand the methods, risks, benefits and alternatives to the study as well as the bearing of these factors on his/her personal clinical situation. Children and adults "with diminished mental capacity" have interests and values regardless of whether they can personally decide whether or not to enroll in a study and this factor must be considered by the investigator and study team.

7. **Respect for potential and enrolled subjects** – Emanuel describes what he calls "Respect for Potential and Enrolled Subjects" and says this principle extends beyond the simple

notion of obtaining and documenting informed consent. He contends that respect must be afforded by study staff to the participant during the entire trial and both before and after. It includes respecting the wishes of the participant to withdraw from the study at any time without fear or reprisal. All personal and private health information about the participant must be protected and confidentiality must be maintained at all times.

Overall, Emanuel and his fellow ethicists conclude that these seven requirements are universal in nature and, thus, pertain to all research studies. They also suggest that if all seven are met that "the vast majority of clinical research" would be deemed ethical. The fulfillment of all seven ensures that research is "socially valuable and subjects are not exploited, that subjects are treated fairly and with respect, and that their interests are protected."

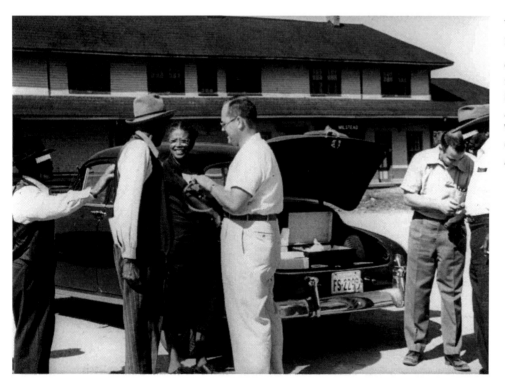

Tuskegee Syphilis Study

eft: unidentified subjects, nurse Eunice Rivers, Dr. David Albritton, and Dr. Walter Edmondson (National Archives-Atlanta, GA)

Summary

Ethical principles and subsequently enacted regulations and laws evolve over time both to adapt to changing science as well as ethical theory and clinical practice. Clear examples include the changes brought about by gene therapy and stem cell research, investigators' financial conflict of interest and life-altering treatments for diseases like HIV-AIDS.

Training and education for all research professionals serve as a requisite for teaching research professionals how to interpret the regulations and can enhance understanding of how to interpret and appropriately apply ethical principles. Over time the interpretation of ethical behavior has changed and our interpretation of the regulations has changed with it. Research participants are best served by research professionals who are mindful of the need to receive ongoing education and training so that they can appropriately apply regulations and ethical principles.

Professional conduct requires us to maintain education and training levels in clinical medicine as well as research ethics. This is particularly true so that we "do no harm", particularly to patients who have voluntarily agreed to enroll in research studies and without whom we would have no clinical research. The oaths that we take as clinicians also challenge us to recognize that conducting clinical research with human subjects is not a right that is bestowed on us with our professional degrees but, rather, a privilege that we must guard on a daily basis.

References

1. US Code of Federal Regulations, 45 CFR 46.

2. US Code of Federal Regulations 21 CFR 50, 21 CFR 56.

3. International Conference on Harmonisation (ICH) E6 Good Clinical Practices

4. "Trials of War Criminals before the Nuremberg Military Tribunals under Control Council Law No. 10, Vol 2, pp. 181-182. Washington, DC: U.S> Government Printing Office, 1949.

5. National Commission for the Protection of Human Subjects of Biomedical and Behavioral Research. *The Belmont Report,* Washington, DC: U.S. Government Printing Office; 1979.

6. 18th World Medical Assembly, Declaration of Helsinki: Ethical Principles for Medical Research Involving Human Subjects. Helsinki, Finland. 1964, amended 1975, 1983, 1989, 1996, 2000 (clarifications added 2002 and 2004).

7. National Commission for the Protection of Human Subjects of Biomedical and Behavioral Research. *The Belmont Report,* Washington, DC: U.S. Government Printing Office; 1979.

8. Jones, JH. *Bad Blood: The Tuskegee Syphilis Experiment.*2nd edition. New York, NY: The Free Press; 1993.

9. Reverby SM,ed.*Tuskegee's Truths: Rethinking the Tuskegee Syphilis Study.* Chapel Hill, NC: University of North Carolina Press; 2000.

10. Directive of December 29, 1900 of the Prussian Minister of Religious, Educational and Medical Affairs addressed to the directors of clinics, polyclinics, and similar establishments (*Centralblatt der gesamten Unterrichtsverwaltung in Preussen,* 1902, pp 188-189). Also see reference 15.

11. "The Guidelines on Innovative Therapy and Scientific Experimentation established by the Circular of February 28, 1931, of the (German) Reich Minister of the interior. (For references see: *Reichgesundheitblatt,*March 11, 1931, No. 10, pp 174-175 and Howard-Jones, "Human Experimentation." Also see reference 15.

12. Levine RJ. Ethics and Regulation of Clinical Research, New Haven, CT, Yale University Press: 1986.

13. Katz J. *Experimentation with Human Beings.* New York, NY: Russell Sage Foundation; 1972.

14. Emanuel EJ, Coruch RA, Arras JD, et al, editors. Ethical and Regulatory aspects of Clinical Research: Readings and Commentary. The Johns Hopkins University Press, Baltimore, Maryland 2003.

15. Annas GJ, Grodin MA. The Nazi Doctors and the Nuremberg Code. New York, NY. Oxford University Press: 1992.

16. Childress JF, Meslin EM, Shapiro HT (editors). Belmont revisited. Washington, DC. Georgetown University Press: 2005.

17. Berg JW, Applebaum PS, Lidz CW, Parker LS (editors). Informed Consent: Legal Theory and Clinical Practice. New York, NY. Oxford University Press: 2001

18. Ellis GB. Keeping Research Subjects Out of Harm's Way. *JAMA*; 2000; 283(20) 2701-2711.

19. Emanuel EJ, Wendler D and Grady C. What Makes Clinical Research Ethical? *JAMA*; 2000;283:(20) 2701-2711.

Chapter 6

The clinical trial process: regulatory affairs

Ms. Sue Green, Shore Ltd.

> Regulatory Affairs is a multi-disciplinary function that acts as the interface between the company and external regulatory bodies.

Introduction – what is regulatory affairs

Clinical trials are externally regulated by both governmental agencies, (regulatory agencies / competent authorities) and ethics committees (ECs) / institutional review boards (IRBs), (may be site specific or national). These bodies are responsible for approving the initiation of a clinical trial and for ensuring that clinical studies are conducted to an appropriate standard in order to safeguard trial participants and protect public safety. The regulatory affairs function provides a bridge between the company and the external regulatory bodies who must approve the design and conduct of a clinical trial in the country concerned. The aim of this chapter is to provide an introduction to the role of regulatory affairs in clinical development and to provide a summary of the main regulatory requirements to be considered when conducting clinical trials.

There is a common misconception that regulatory affairs provide a 'policing' role within a company: dotting the i's and crossing the t's to ensure that a company stays within certain boundaries. The role of a modern regulatory professional is however, much more dynamic and interactive. The regulatory function is multidisciplinary and should be an integrated part of the product development team in order to provide timely advice and to have input into the overall development strategy and timelines.

> The regulatory affairs function provides a bridge between the company and the external regulatory bodies who must approve the design and conduct of a clinical trial.

Regulatory professionals have an overall knowledge and understanding of the local regulatory procedures and data requirements. They advise the team as to the level of quality, chemistry, manufacturing & controls (CMC), non-clinical and clinical data required to support an application to conduct a clinical trial at each phase of development and are responsible for the compilation and submission of clinical trial / investigational new drug applications (CTA's / IND's) in the required territories.

Regulatory affairs act as the interface between the company and the regulators with whom they will have a working relationship which enables them to actively follow the progress of applications, receive, discuss and respond to questions raised and arrange and conduct face to face meetings between the company and the regulators as required. The group will also provide advice on the implementation of any amendments to a trial and ensure that the necessary external approvals are in place to support any changes, thus protecting the integrity of a trial while avoiding costly delays or interruptions to the conduct of the trial itself.

A good regulatory affairs professional should have a comprehensive understanding of the product development plan and therapeutic area and therefore be in a position to provide input to the development team as to the design and number of trials required to provide data to support the registration of the target product profile in a particular territory, e.g. the need for an active comparator arm to support European Union licensure or the stratification of patients according to severity of disease. The regulatory group will have access to the relevant national guidelines to ensure that local standards and the expectations of external agencies are met, thus minimizing delays, e.g., the need for reproductive toxicity data prior to the inclusion of women of childbearing potential into a clinical study. In addition to having responsibility for the compilation of the required core submission dossiers which provide summaries of the quality, non-clinical and clinical data available on a product (e.g. Investigational New Drug (IND) product dossier in the US or the Investigational Medicinal Product (IMP) dossier in the EU), the regulatory function should also have input into the preparation and approval of a number of documents generated to support a clinical trial application such as the investigators brochure, clinical and non-clinical protocols and labeling, thereby ensuring consistency in approach and documentation.

> A good regulatory affairs professional should have a comprehensive understanding of the product development plan and therapeutic area.

Why is regulatory affairs needed?

The regulatory function has both a strategic and functional role in drug development, providing strategic advice on the design and implementation of a product development plan and having the knowledge and expertise to prepare and maintain the necessary submissions to the local health authorities

Strategic role

Regulatory affairs is needed strategically to ensure that the team is aware of any local clinical and regulatory requirements associated with the development of a particular medicinal product for a target indication in a given territory. They should inform the team of any new developments / regulatory requirements which could affect the manufacturing development or clinical program thereby minimizing any delays in product development, e.g. allowing for additional data requirements for first-in-man studies and advising the team if the investigational medicinal product is likely to be subject to special measures.

As a proactive and integrated part of the product development team, global regulatory affairs advise on the relevant guidelines and agency standards, which may apply when taking a particular product from first principles, through a clinical trial program to registration. In the context of clinical trials the regulatory function plays a pivotal role in identifying regulatory milestones, which should be met in order to ensure a smooth approval process. Regulatory affairs should be able to provide guidance on the level of information required by the external agencies to support the conduct of the proposed trial and to quantify the risks associated with providing a different data package to that expected by the regulatory bodies, e.g. restriction of patient population in a clinical trial may have implications on the final product label approved.

Functional role

The regulatory function is needed to prepare, submit and maintain the clinical trial applications in concerned territories. While the majority of territories use a common IMP dossier template for submissions, this is a common format and not common content and given the large amount of legislation in place to protect patients and the plethora of regional and therapeutic guidelines to be considered, regional regulatory experts are important to provide further information on the local regulatory requirements in the geographic region of interest; in the USA, for example, full study reports are usually required to support the non-clinical summary, whereas most other regulatory agencies accept summary data only. Indeed, while a global product development team often has one regulatory representative to provide strategic input into the overall development plan and to prepare the master documentation, local regulatory representatives are often used to prepare and submit the trial applications in the target territories as they have specialized local regulatory knowledge and a good relationship with their relevant health authorities.

Regulatory affairs act as the interface between the company and the health authorities and will be the contact point for regulatory agencies assessing the trial applications. They will help to interpret requests from authorities and assess any impact such requests could have on the clinical trial, such as the need for protocol amendments (which may need submitting in other participating countries). All communications and requests from agencies should be discussed with the project team, as decisions should not be made locally, even to minor requests from health authorities as this could affect the overall integrity of the trial.

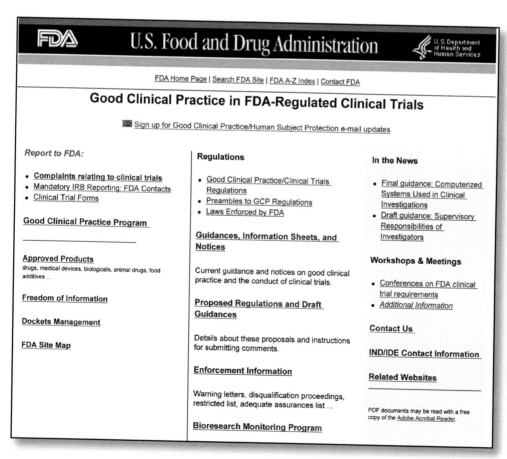

"Many regulatory agencies have comprehensive and well-maintained websites providing comprehensive and regularly updated information to sponsors."

The external regulatory environment

The external regulatory environment is influenced by several factors including international guidelines, (such as ICH), national legislation, available local guidelines, (which may be related to the target therapeutic area or class of product), local treatment practice and historical precedent. This is further complicated in Europe where there are both EU and national regulations, directives and guidelines to be taken into account. The clinical trial directive (Directive 2001/20/EC), for example is an EU directive that was released in Europe in 2001 and contains recommendations regarding the approval process for the conduct of clinical trials within the EU. All EU countries were required to incorporate the rules of the directive into national legislation by 2003 and to put this into effect by 2004 but each country had the autonomy to interpret the recommendations when incorporating them into national law. Accordingly, national requirements and processes for clinical trial applications vary from country to country within the EU member states. Conversely in the US, section 21 part 312 of the Code of Federal Regulations (21CFR 312) legislates for all investigational new drug applications in the USA and whilst additional guidances are available for certain types of investigational drug, clinical trials and target therapy areas, these are governed by the same federal legislation outlined in 21CFR 312.

Regulatory affairs should evaluate all of these factors and ensure that all available information is taken into account by the team when designing a clinical development program. First-in-man studies are commonly conducted within one or two territories as they typically involve small patient numbers and specialist Phase I units, but clinical trials enacted later in the development program are usually conducted in a number of international territories. It is not uncommon to find that the recommended endpoints and patient population for trials in a target therapeutic area vary from territory to territory particularly when designing an international clinical program spanning Europe, the USA and Australasia. It is therefore important to fully understand the background to the relevant requirements and be able to interpret and adapt these in order to design a clinical development program, which will support international registration of the target label.

There are two types of 'regulatory bodies' involved in the review and approval of clinical trials, 1) regional health authorities, (also known as the competent authorities) and 2) ethics committees / institutional review boards. Applications must be made to both of these bodies and approval obtained from each prior to the initiation of a clinical trial.

Competent authorities

The competent authorities are the regional health authorities / regulatory agencies. These are governmental agencies responsible for the regulation and control of the use of investigational medicinal products. Each country has its own regulatory agency and national approval process for clinical trial applications, which are specific to that individual country. In the USA trial applications may be reviewed by one of two bodies within the Food and Drug Agency (FDA), the Center for Drug Evaluation and Research (CDER) or the Center for Biologics Evaluation and Research (CBER), the body reviewing the application being dependant upon the nature of the investigational medicinal product to be studied in clinical trials. Although there may be some differences in IND data requirements due to the nature of the product, both CDER and CBER are subject to the provisions set out in 21CFR 312 and work to a common process. In the EU however, contrary to the situation for marketed products, the European Medicines Agency (EMEA) is not involved in reviewing and approving EU trial applications and each EU Country has its own regulatory agency responsible for the assessment of clinical trial applications, which are subject to their national laws and approval processes.

> It is important to have local regulatory professionals responsible for the submission of local dossiers.

The regulatory affairs function is usually responsible for the preparation and submission of clinical trial applications to competent authorities and is the contact point for any queries / dialogue on the submission. While English is commonly accepted as the language for the 'investigational medicinal product,' (IMP) dossier used throughout Europe, local application forms, country specific documentation and the cover letter must be written in the local language. It is important therefore, to have local regulatory professionals responsible for the submission of local dossiers and dialogue with assessors.

Clinical trial applications made to competent authorities are processed in accordance with a pre-determined timeframe; (A 30 day review cycle applies in the USA, whereas in Europe the clinical trial directive mandates that applications to competent authorities must be assessed within a total of 60 days). Procedures for review within national agencies vary, however, and many competent authorities also have an additional pre-submission and validation phase. This should be taken into account when planning clinical trials. Furthermore, some competent authorities have additional regulatory bodies which are responsible for the review of clinical trial applications for certain products e.g. applications for trials using products of biotechnology must reviewed by the viral safety committee in France and the RIVM (National Institute for Public Health and the Environment) in the Netherlands in addition to the competent authority review. In these cases multiple applications are required to satisfy the competent authority and the timelines for the submission and review of such applications should be factored into the clinical development plan.

Ethics Committees (ECs) / Institutional Review Boards (IRBs)

Ethics committees (EU) or institutional review boards (USA) are independent bodies consisting of scientists, healthcare professionals and non-medical members whose responsibility is to protect the rights, safety and well-being of human subjects involved in a clinical trial. Approval from these committees is required in order to conduct a clinical trial in a given country. These boards are usually linked to a hospital or research facility involved in the conduct of the clinical trial and it reviews patient and study specific documentation such as the investigators brochure, study protocol, informed consent forms, insurance etc although the level of documentation required varies according to individual committees. Given that ethics committees and IRBs are associated with clinical operations, submissions to these committees are usually managed by the clinical team and are not considered to be the responsibility of the regulatory group, indeed in some countries the submission to the ethics committee must be made by the principal investigator involved in the study rather than by the company.

Ethics committees / IRBs meet according to a pre-defined schedule and therefore the timing of the submission of clinical trial applications must be carefully managed. The majority of ethics committees accept submissions in parallel with those made to the competent authority, although some still require evidence of health authority approval prior to issuing a favourable opinion. Given that the timing for review and approval of an ethics submission is similar to that of the submission to the competent authority and that both applications are often progressing in parallel, it is essential that there is a good working relationship within the different functions in the company responsible for managing the submission.

Meeting international standards

Global harmonization efforts have been ongoing within the pharmaceutical industry since the unification of Europe in the 1980s. This led to the generation of the European Medicines Agency (EMEA), pan European guidelines and the elaboration of the European Pharmacopoeia (Ph.Eur). These attempts at harmonization were further extended with the formation of the International Conference of Harmonisation (ICH) in 1990, which involved industry and agency representatives from Europe, USA and Japan coming together to review the requirements for product registration in order to agree upon common principles and standards which should apply during drug development. The aim of ICH was to make recommendations for harmonization in order to obviate the need for duplicate testing of medicinal products. Accordingly, national agencies have established their own recommendations and procedures for the approval and conduct of clinical trials as described previously. These are underpinned by common international principles and standards such as good clinical practice and the use of MedDRA coding (Medical Dictionary for Regulatory Affairs) for the classification of adverse events. (See box on following page for further discussion.)

> ICH was to make recommendations for harmonization in order to obviate the need for duplicate testing of medicinal products.

The format of trial documentation has also been standardized with the issue of ICH E3 providing guidance on the structure and content of clinical study reports, the implementation of the EU clinical trial directive and generation of ICH M4, the ICH common technical document (CTD). The CTD was originally generated to provide a

International regulatory harmonization

Different events in the US, Europe and Japan led to the idea that an independent evaluation of medicinal products was necessary prior to them being allowed on the market. However, this process remained nationally-based and over time did not reflect the growing international nature of the pharmaceutical industry's activities. Thus, much of the regulatory process was being repeated in each of the markets, which led to delays in launching products that would serve an unmet medical need and unnecessary expense and use of resources in satisfying each regulatory agency's requirements. Since the 1990s, there has been a move to harmonize the regulatory requirements in different world regions.

Often referred to as simply ICH, the International Conference on Harmonisation of Technical Requirements for Registration of Pharmaceuticals for Human Use (ICH) is a unique initiative that seeks to promote greater regulatory harmony between different world regions. Specifically, ICH brings together the regulatory authorities of Europe, Japan and the United States and experts from the pharmaceutical industry in these three regions to discuss scientific and technical aspects of product registration.

ICH is composed of six parties that represent the regulatory bodies and research-based industry in the US, European Union and Japan:

✦ In the US, the members are the Food and Drug Administration (FDA), and the Pharmaceutical Research and Manufacturers of America (PhRMA)

✦ In Europe, the members are the European Union (EU), and the European Federation of Pharmaceutical Industries and Associations (EFPIA)

✦ In Japan, the members are the Ministry of Health, Labour and Welfare (MHLW), and the Japan Pharmaceutical Manufacturers Association (JPMA)

In addition, ICH has Observers that represent non-ICH countries and regions. These are the World Health Organization (WHO), Health Canada, and the European Free Trade Association (EFTA).

ICH is operated via the ICH Steering Committee, which is supported by ICH Coordinators and the ICH Secretariat, based in Switzerland. The Steering Committee governs the ICH, determines its policies and procedures, selects topics for harmonization and monitors the progress of harmonization initiatives. Each of the six ICH parties has two seats on the ICH Steering Committee. Each of the Observers nominates non-voting participants to attend the ICH Steering Committee Meetings. The International Federation of Pharmaceutical Manufacturers and Associations (IFPMA), which represents the pharmaceutical industry at an international level, also participates as a non-voting member.

By achieving consensus, recommendations can be made to improve the processes for product registration and thereby reduce the need for duplicative testing in each region that might otherwise have been required during the research and development of new medicines. Harmonization allows the better use of resources in developing new medicines and also reduces the delay in bringing new drugs to the patients that need them.

ICH also serves as a focus point to maintain safeguards on quality, safety and efficacy, and regulatory obligations to protect public health. ICH harmonization involves a step-wise progression of guidelines, various maintenance activities, as well as processes to modify existing guidelines and assist in their implementation. The topics that ICH discusses are divided into four main categories: Quality, Safety, Efficacy and Multidisciplinary (Table 1).

Table 1: ICH discussion topics

ICH Topics	Details
Quality	Relates to chemical and pharmaceutical quality assurance.
Safety	Relates to in vitro and in vivo pre-clinical studies
Efficacy	Relates to clinical studies in human subjects
Multidisciplinary	Relates to cross-cutting topics which do not fit uniquely into one of the above categories

framework for license applications, and its format has been largely adopted for clinical trial applications. The majority of international countries now accept clinical trial applications in this format. Although this does not remove regional differences in content, it avoids unnecessary reformatting of data to different territories and allows for the regulatory group within a company to prepare and maintain a central master document on the investigational medicinal product. This document can then be further adapted for individual territories.

When creating international clinical trial applications it is important to remember that although there are commonly accepted formats and principles, the content of an application is not always harmonized between countries. Investigational medicinal products being studied in trials in Europe must meet the quality standards set out in the European pharmacopeia whereas trials conducted in the US or Japan may only use materials that have been tested and released according to their national pharmacopoeial standards (USP and JP, respectively). Most materials meet multi-pharmacopoeial standards, however, this can lead to additional testing. For example, water for injection (WFI), which is commonly used in the manufacture of pharmaceuticals, has different accepted methods of manufacture in the EU compared to the US. Furthermore, as the efforts of ICH have concentrated on gaining consensus on registration requirements for pharmaceuticals there still remain differences as to when data should be generated during the clinical development program. Reproductive toxicity testing is a good example of this divergence. EU authorities generally require some embryo-fetal toxicity testing to be conducted prior to the inclusion of women of childbearing potential in clinical studies, whereas these data are not required until Phase III in the US, and must be generated prior to the initiation of a clinical trial program in Japan. Regulatory Affairs should advise the team as to these national variations as they can have a major impact on the conduct of a clinical trial program.

The most common areas of diversity, however, are related to national submission procedure and local clinical practice. In the US, there is a close working relationship between the company and the authority (FDA) with pre-submission meetings and on-going dialogue encouraged, whereas in the EU such close interactions may not always be possible, particularly during the review process as trial applications are managed by national agencies who are trying to adhere to the standard review times set out in the clinical trial directive. Following the problems encountered in the Phase I study with TeGenero's TGN-1412 (See box overleaf), revisions to the requirements for first-in-man studies have been implemented across Europe and pre-submission meetings such as those held with the FDA prior to the submission of an IND are now recommended.

Divergence in international clinical practice is due to a number of factors. Between Europe, the US and Australasia, the body responsible for the funding of healthcare has a major influence on clinical practice. In the US, healthcare is largely privately funded whereas in Europe and Australasia the costs are mainly borne by the government. These differences are compounded by the fact that the US is mainly a large homogenous country with respect to healthcare funding and opinion leader bodies whereas the EU remains heterogenous with differences in government funding mechanisms, the proportion of government funding, and healthcare policies. Furthermore, each nation has its own opinion leader bodies generating national treatment guidelines for key areas of medicine.

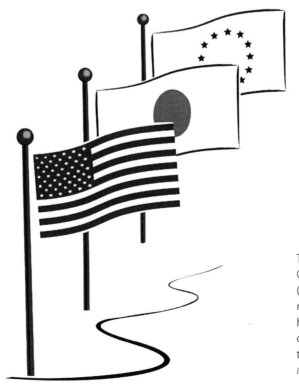

The aim of International Conference of Harmonisation (ICH) was to make recommendations for harmonization in order to obviate the need for duplicate testing of medicinal products.

Illustration by Wadi Talhami, NY

Adverse incidents during the clinical trial of TeGenero TGN1412

A clinical trial that generated substantial publicity in the media and focused attention on regulatory agencies was the first-in-human study of the monoclonal antibody TGN1412, a compound developed by the German biotech company, TeGenero AG. The trial was conducted for TeGenero by Parexel, a large contract research organization at its hospital-based facility in North London, UK. Eight healthy male volunteers were recruited and dosed on March 13, 2006. After receiving injections of TGN1412, six of the volunteers became seriously ill, had multiple organ failure and were transferred to an intensive care unit. According to Parexel, the subjects experienced "Cytokine Release Syndrome", which was reported as "life-threatening". Although the volunteers were eventually discharged from the hospital, the outlook for their future health has been described as uncertain and this has led to an ongoing legal action against those who conducted the study.

The unexpected and serious outcome of the TGN1412 trial led to investigations under the supervision of the UK's Medicines and Healthcare products Regulatory Agency (MHRA), which had originally approved the trial and its protocol. Other European authorities also became involved in the subsequent investigations.

The Tegenero case led to regulatory agencies around the world re-evaluating their procedures, with particular emphasis on how to conduct first-in-man studies for high-risk monoclonal antibodies and other therapeutic proteins. The case has also had implications for initiatives involving collaboration between regulators and pharmaceutical companies. For example, although it was not set up specifically for this case, a number of pharmaceutical companies are members of the Predictive Safety Testing Consortium, where they will share information previously considered commercially sensitive in an attempt to better predict how new experimental drugs will work in the human body. This project has been co-ordinated as part of the FDA's Critical Path Initiative (C-Path), a major project aiming to streamline drug discovery and research.

These divergences in practice are emphasized by the widely different uptake of innovative medicines across the different markets and lead to difficulty in defining a common 'gold standard of care' for a given therapy area. Regulatory professionals should evaluate these differences and advise on the design of clinical studies required to support the overall positioning of the product and minimize any negative impact on the registration of the target label in different territories. The design of the trial is not simply related to the choice of active comparator for product positioning however, as importantly the EU authorities generally require active comparator studies (using the current gold standard for treatment), to be conducted to support licensure in Europe, whereas the US usually request that confirmatory studies are placebo controlled. Discussions with the regulatory agencies concerned are therefore paramount prior to the initiation of these studies in order to design a mutually acceptable international clinical program, which supports registration of the target label. The regulatory function are responsible for the initiation, preparation and conduct of such discussions and should advice the team as to appropriate timelines for agency meetings in order to avoid delays in the clinical development program.

Summary and conclusion

In summary, Regulatory Affairs is a multi-disciplinary function that acts as the interface between the company and external regulatory bodies. They have an overall knowledge of regulatory processes, international standards and data requirements for the conduct and initiation of clinical studies and advise the team on the format, content and timing of clinical trial applications to the relevant regulatory bodies. Regulatory Affairs have overall responsibility for generating and submitting trial applications and for managing communications with local regulatory agencies.

The regulatory role is a dynamic and interactive one which provides a bridge between product development and registration by assisting the project team in designing a clinical development plan that can take a product from first concept to registration of the target label (and beyond).

When designing and conducting a clinical development plan consideration should be given to the following regulatory milestones:

- ✦ Overall product positioning and target label
- ✦ Local clinical practices including identification of 'gold standard' of care
- ✦ Target patient population
- ✦ Data requirements to support the timely initiation of clinical studies
- ✦ International standards
- ✦ Generation of a central core Investigational Medicinal Product (IMP) / Investigational New Drug (IND) dossier
- ✦ Local regulatory requirements
- ✦ Timing of applications to competent authorities and EC/IRBs
- ✦ Identification of regional differences (and consideration as to how these can be met without impacting the overall development plan)
- ✦ Meetings with regulatory authorities.

References

1. International Conference on Harmonisation of Technical Requirements for Registration of Pharmaceuticals for Human Use (ICH). http://www.ich.org

2. Wood AJ and Darbyshire J (2006).Injury to research volunteers--the clinical-research nightmare. N Engl J Med. 2006 May 4;354(18):1869-71.

3. MHRA (2006). Investigations into adverse incidents during clinical trials of TGN1412. Medicines and Healthcare products Regulatory Agency (MHRA). 25 May 2006. http://www.mhra.gov.uk

4. Anon (2006). Companies share secrets to reduce unforeseen phase I problems. PharmaFocus 26 April 2006. http://www.pharmafocus.com/cda/focusH/1,2109,21-0-0-APR_2006-focus_news_detail-0-436916,00.html

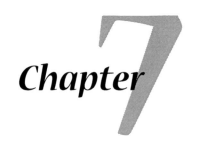

Chapter 7

The clinical trial process: monitoring

Dr. Ignazio Di Giovanna, HonFICR, CCA 2000 Ltd

Dr. Gareth Hayes, HonFICR, Phlexglobal Ltd

Good monitoring will lead
to a good study.

Introduction

So you're a CRA, a Clinical Trials Monitor…a Clinical Trials Coordinator…Clinical Scientist…whatever the title one thing is true, you will at sometime or other, carry out monitoring of clinical trial data. So what's it all about and why is it possibly the most important part of the whole clinical trial process? Why does monitoring data provide the cornerstone of a good clinical study?

To be a good monitor you need to be a detail-obsessed-schizophrenic…you need to be a scientist, a psychologist, a data processor, memory-person, be able to listen to two people at the same time while rolling the protocol around your brain to sift out that one vital line which will help you justify why the patient should not have been included, a motivator…and as if that's not enough, you'll sometimes also need to be a sympathetic ear and counselor.

The whole clinical development process for investigational products is highly regulated. The Monitor plays a crucial role in ensuring adherence to these regulations during the clinical trial.

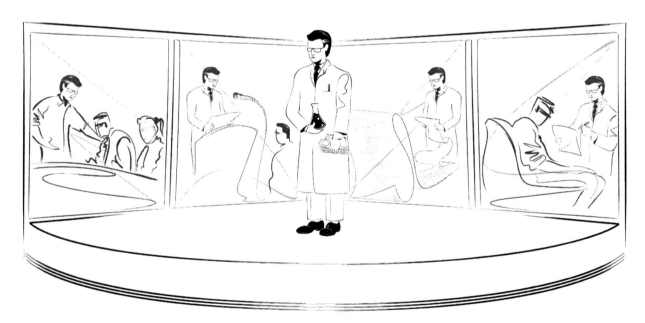

Multitasking is fundamental to being a good monitor.

Illustration by Wadi Talhami, NY

By definition, monitoring is the part of the trial during which the Active Phase of patient (or subject) recruitment and treatment takes place. A monitor's job is essentially to represent the Sponsor and ensure that the patients/subjects selected for a study are appropriate, and that they have consented and have undergone all relevant protocol related study procedures. Monitors must also ensure that the data collected by an investigational site is truthful, accurate, clear and unambiguous.

Good monitoring will lead to a good study, a high level of confidence in the data collected and ultimately a good study report. Bad or mediocre monitoring will result in, at the very least, a high rate of data queries (depending on the center's experience, of course) to at the very worst and extreme, repeated enrolment of unsuitable patients and erroneous and or dubious data collection, delays in time to data base lock and time to study report.

Good and effective monitoring therefore ensures that the study is run to the appropriate legal, ethical, moral and safety standards and therefore helps to safeguard the interests and well being of clinical study subjects.

The project team's critical path analysis reveals many Key Performance Measures (KPMs) during a trial's lifetime from protocol development to final report, but there is no doubt that the monitoring function is the most vital. And as these KPMs define to the hour that "time is money" it becomes all the more apparent how important an effective monitor is to success, and to proving the oxymoron that is high quality at high speed.

The monitor's responsibilities vary in length and detail. The extent to which a monitor is involved in the clinical trial process depends very much on the individual's ability, experience and background. It also depends on the company and its management structure. Hence, in small organizations a monitor may take a study from brief concept, protocol development, development of supporting documentation, site selection, study initiation, study monitoring, closure of study center, study report writing and possibly even presentation of the results. Whereas, in larger organizations each of these functions (and some other intervening functions) may well be performed by separate groups of dedicated individuals.

The clinical trial process

The clinical trial process can be considered in terms of a good book or novel, with a start, middle and end. So, at the start the scene is set and the main characters are introduced, following which the plot develops, invariably taking a number of twists and turns, finally the plot is revealed leading to a clear and final end…or to the cliff hanger…with uncertainty and begging for a sequel. In clinical trial terms we therefore have;

- ✦ *Setting the scene*: study set-up and initiation,
- ✦ *Developing the plot*: clinical (active) phase; subject recruitment and treatment
- ✦ *The reveal*: study close and report.

Study setup and initiation

A pre-study visit must be made to each study site (or center) to assess the suitability of the investigators and facilities and to discuss in detail the requirements of the study, including regulatory requirements, the ethics committee review and remuneration. The pre-study visit can be considered one of the most important visits, as the selection of a suitable investigator and site ultimately can dictate the success of the study. The pre-study visit may not be one single visit but a series of visits. For example, it may not be logistically possible to meet all site personnel, pharmacy and laboratory staff at one time. The pre-study visits can be divided into three distinct sections: investigator selection, site suitability and items concerning overall study conduct.

Investigator selection

It is essential to gain information about the investigator's general experience in the field and more specifically with clinical trials, including previous experience of working to Good Clinical Practice (GCP) standards; check that the investigator has sufficient time to conduct the study to the standards required and ensure that the investigator has an adequate subject population for the trial. The investigators' curriculum vitae documents should be concise and fully up to date and show that they are appropriately qualified.

Site suitability

Site staff must have appropriate qualifications and experience to perform the study and undertake the study procedures, and have no conflict of time and of interest. A site's facilities, both in terms of space and equipment, must be adequate and appropriate for the study.

> The monitors must ensure that the investigator understands their responsibilities.

Study conduct

An investigator must have a full understanding of the protocol and be aware of his study obligations. The monitor 'shares' these obligations by reinforcing through discussion the provisions and requirements for the independent ethics committee (IEC/IRB) and for informed consent. The monitor must discuss all aspects of study conduct with the investigator such as review of administrative aspects, including remuneration, direct access to source documents, timing of the study with start and end dates, procedures for study monitoring and the requirement for the storage of data at the end of the study as well as procedures for all aspects of drug accountability. The monitor must ensure that the investigator understands their responsibilities for all personnel to whom they delegate responsibilities, also that they have a full understanding of the protocol, and what part they are expected to take in the study and in helping the investigator to fulfill his or her study obligations.

Investigator meetings

During the pre-study phase it is usual to hold a meeting of the investigators and support staff to provide training on the drug, study procedures, requirements of GCP guidelines and all aspects of the trial. The meeting must act as a forum for communication, information and motivation. The monitor comes into his or her own here, as driver for the whole project. This is the meeting where, by gaining buy-in, the monitor sells the study and introduces team spirit and shared goals.

Site initiation

Study initiation at the site is a monitoring task only conducted when the investigator and study site have been approved and all clinical trial supplies are available. The visit purpose is to ensure a full comprehension of the study by all who are involved in the study and that all essential documents have been collected and validated for regulatory assurance. Both during and following the monitoring visit the monitor should make appropriate notes as a formal record of the visit. This will usually be done on a pre-designed report form. The monitor can use such templates as aids to monitoring but they must be aware that they still have to think rather than perform the exercises as 'tick-box' activities.

Clinical phase

Study monitoring visits

How often the monitor has to be on-site or visiting the investigator is nearly always more than they can actually physically achieve, even if they had endless resource and budget. The frequency of routine monitoring visits will clearly depend upon the complexity of the study, the phase of the study and the treatment period. What is apparent is that the early stages of a study are critical and the first monitoring visit should take place either following treatment of the first few subjects or after the first assessments have been made. As a general rule, and it is only a general rule, monitoring visits will occur more frequently for Phase I and Phase II studies - every 2–6 weeks – than for larger Phase III and IV studies - every 4-8 weeks – where time frames and treatment periods are likely to be longer and safety measurements more assured (but no less important). The "double it and again" principle when considering timelines and subject recruitment rates is used by experienced study managers. In other words, rarely will the monitor be able to keep to strict visit times. Subject (patient) recruitment rates are also rarely what's hoped for at the start of the study. However, every best effort can be made and visit dates should at least be planned well in advance by careful, and disciplined, use of the diary. There is no reason why all the visit dates for a particular site cannot be put in the diary (of both monitor and investigator) at the start of the study. In our experience this has never happened and, if at has, then within a few days the wall planner is ripped from the wall as dates are pushed back and days become full.

Time management and organizational skills are a prerequisite of the monitor's skill set. The monitor must devote sufficient time to planning and preparation of each and every site visit. The reason for the visit should not be as unspecific as "monitoring visit due" and the phrase 'it's in the detail' suddenly becomes the monitor's motto. Perhaps the reason for the visit would be to *"check recent* Case Record Forms" (CRFs) and *"collect outstanding data"* as a priority, with *"update staff on progress"* and *"check drug accountability logs"* as examples of other objectives.

Safety and adverse events

"Safety of Medicines" is a core obligation of all our studies and the monitor must be alert to all aspects of safety monitoring. Trial protocols detail the methodology of recording and reporting adverse events, including by whom and to whom and how efficiently reports must be submitted. Significantly, it is during the active recruiting phase of the study that, sometimes, only the monitor will be able to see the arising incidences of adverse events across the trial. A good monitor, while addressing true confidentiality from subject's identification, may find themselves closer to the study and its data by being more aware of each subject as they progress through the trial. At each routine monitoring visit the monitor must scrupulously review all the adverse events documented in the case report form in line with the protocol and monitoring guidelines. The monitor, who falls under the auspices of the investigator, must be alert for serious adverse events, interpretations of severity across assessments, and the due reporting responsibilities.

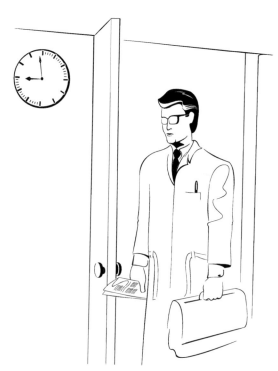

The frequency of routine monitoring visits will clearly depend upon the complexity of the study. *Illustration by Wadi Talhami, NY*

Laboratory, pharmacy and other key contacts

In studies involving a clinical laboratory, the monitor needs to have an understanding of routine hematology and biochemistry tests, whether this is sampling techniques or expected results bearing in mind therapeutic challenge or variations due to the subject's indications. The recent use of tissue sampling for genetic research has a continuing impact on ethical issues, and is seen by many to be revolutionizing health outcomes. Monitors may find themselves clarifying many questions on this subject from investigators, study staff and, indeed, indirectly, the subjects. The assessment of drug accountability and reconciliation, combined with subject compliance is one of the most crucial parts of a monitor's duties and this will involve a positive relationship with the dispensing pharmacy or clinical trials pharmacist.

> [O]nly the monitor will be able to see the arising incidences of adverse events across the trial.

Real monitoring!

The monitor has a responsibility to thoroughly check CRFs for completeness, accuracy, consistency, and credibility. Data validation of this type is a meticulous and time consuming activity best suited to a quiet environment with few or no interruptions. It is difficult to check CRFs in a busy, cramped environment but this may often be the case and the monitor must employ a tidy, structured system. Note taking and list making are essential in the cross referencing process. The majority of corrections made to CRF data are because of clarification requirements and this can become frustrating for the monitor, investigator and site staff. It can also impinge on the accuracy of reporting of 'clean' data, simply because of paperwork and undue workload. Patience and diplomacy, combined with authoritative persistence, early in the study can prevent repeated paper chases and reduce error risk. Sponsor companies use a variety of query log forms and monitors must work closely with the Statisticians and Data Management units to ensure shared familiarity and consistency. The completion of the data validation CRF checking process is validated in its own way by completion of relevant monitoring logs or assessment sheets. Monitors will be expected to confirm and clarify key efficacy and safety data on CRFs

The monitoring visit

✓ Review and re-review the facilities, equipment and resources.

✓ Check staff lists for changes and collect signatures of new staff authorized to complete CRFs. Ensure that they are fully updated on trial conduct and procedures.

✓ Review completed CRFs. Cross-reference the CRF data against source documents.

✓ Take action regarding query resolution by bringing discrepancies to the attention of the investigator or clinical team for appropriate resolution

✓ Check current status of subject recruitment including the number of subjects ongoing, completed and withdrawn from the study.

✓ Check recruitment consistency between the CRF count, investigator understanding, and other sources, such as laboratory or pharmacy.

✓ Thoroughly check all information relating to subjects with adverse events and cross-reference with other documentation, e.g. laboratory results, diary cards.

✓ Thoroughly check all information relating to withdrawn subjects and cross-reference with other documentation, e.g. laboratory results, diary cards.

✓ Confirm that protocol amendments have correctly been dealt with, identify protocol violations, and take action as appropriate.

✓ Review subject consent forms for completion and validity by cross-referencing against visit dates and signatories.

✓ Check drug accountability and cross reference with dispensing logs. Take action for collection and/or disposal of returned unused medication and confirm that trial supplies are suitably stocked.

✓ Contact other departments, e.g. laboratory, and conduct relevant checks and updates.

✓ For blinded studies, check the emergency code break procedure status and take relevant action regarding code breaks.

✓ Review any issues since the last visit or unresolved issues since the last contact.

✓ Check the completeness, accuracy and integrity of the Investigator Site File.

✓ Make an appointment for the next visit.

✓ Fully document each visit!

against source documents and also require the rigorous checking of data involving, dates of visits, consent details, eligibility, drug accountability and more. Cross-referencing will include laborious tasks such as checking the correct subject number appears on each CRF and associated documentation. Clinical or medical aptitude may not be an expected qualification of the Monitor, yet a related expertise in observation is necessary to be an effective monitor. Monitors should be able to 'monitor' matters of clinical importance as the study proceeds rather than at the time of study analysis.

Study close-out

Close-out monitoring visits

Study closure at a site, much as the initiation visit, usually takes more than one visit. If the previous monitoring visits have been meticulously carried out the close-out visit will be a formality. Nevertheless, it is essential to retain the rigorous discipline of previous visits as anomalies and points of clarification will inevitably occur.

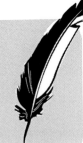

> [E]xpertise in observation is necessary to be an effective monitor.

The close-out or termination visit can also occur when an investigator or site stops, or is stopped, before the course of the trial is run. This can be for a number of reasons, from poor recruitment to change of circumstances. In any case, it is a situation likely to need utmost diplomacy from the monitor. An investigator with interests and priorities lying elsewhere may have little motivation to help complete the formal close-out procedures. By and large the investigator will be grateful to the monitor for helping 'tidy-up' the study at the end and it is important to leave the site with all parties highly motivated and pleased with the work.

Monitoring skills and capabilities

Interpersonal skills are as important as the intellectual skills required for the role of effective monitor. The monitor has to be self-starting, using initiative alongside abilities for multitasking. The monitor's approach is key to efficient study setup and successful subject recruitment. Essential interpersonal skills include diplomacy, negotiation, problem solving and effective communication. Both verbal and non-verbal communication styles are needed throughout the study and especially during the active monitoring phase. Knowing when to be firm as well as being able to use compassion are facets of effective communication.

The monitor should always appear professional, organized and business-like. Self-confidence and enthusiasm are important and continual encouragement and motivation will ensure that any study issues should be resolved quickly and efficiently. Strength of character is paramount. A tough skin and an ability to stand your ground are good virtues. Versatility and flexibility has to be maintained, as sudden reorganization is common in both the pharmaceutical industry and across the healthcare environment in general.

> **Interpersonal skills are as important as the intellectual skills required for the role of effective monitor.**

The monitor has to have the intuitive character of a motivator and leader, yet show the discipline of someone who is stringently methodical and shows a great attention to detail. The monitor must possess a natural energy that is exhibited as an enthusiastic drive, supported by strong ethical values. Regarding the monitor's skill portfolio, many companies now provide a list of competencies essential for the monitor role. Listed competencies will naturally include the knowledge and skills and tasks mentioned above. These tasks can often be linked to Standard Operating Procedures (SOPs) and as such these make suitable reference points.

Summary and conclusion

The role of the monitor can be one of the most varied in the disciplines concerned with pharmaceutical research and development. It is essential that the monitor be efficient with time management and prioritization. A monitor needs to be assertive with the investigator and honest with his study manager from the start. An extra hour spent at the start of the study may end up saving a day at the end. Communication skills should be employed throughout the study to clarify any arising issues for prompt resolution and prevention of reoccurrence. Patience and meticulous record keeping must be employed when dealing with documentation. Some predictive capabilities will allow positive use of sharing best practice and damage limitation; in other words, experience can be the best attribute of a monitor.

References and recommended reading

To be a CRA, Information on the role of a Clinical Research Associate; The Institute of Clinical Research, ISBN 0-9549345-4-7, 2005

Clinical Research Manual, Edited by David Luscombe and Peter D Stonier, Euromed Communications Ltd, ISSN 1355-4808, 2005

Careers with the Pharmaceutical Industry, Edited by Peter D Stonier, John Wiley and Sons, ISBN 0-470-84328-4, 2003

Principles of Clinical Research, Edited by Ignazio Di Giovanna and Gareth Hayes, Wrightson Biomedical Publishing Ltd., ISBN 1-871816-45-9, 2001.

Chapter 8

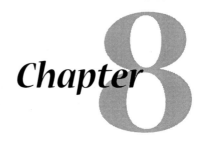

The clinical trial process: statistics

Ms. Cathy O'Brien, Fincham Statistics Ltd

Statistics are used to test
the hypothesis.

Introduction

In an ideal 'uniform' world, we would all reach adulthood with the same height, weight and appearance. We might make allowances and suggest that women were 10 cm shorter than men, but generally in this 'ideal' world all adults would have the same metabolism, heart rate, blood pressure and life would be quite boring. In reality, we all end up with different shapes and sizes, and although there will be some very tall people and some very short people, most people will be within certain limits of the average height, as illustrated below.

Cumulative probability plot for height (average = 178cm, SD = 5cm)

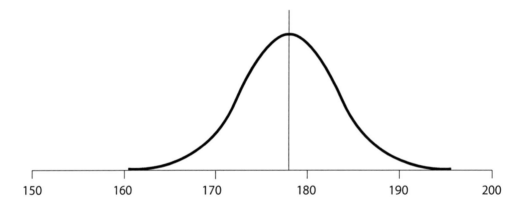

The same is true when it comes to being treated; there are few medications that can provide instantaneous relief from an ailment. Even when a treatment does offer a cure, all patients will not respond in the same way. It will take different lengths of time, or a different number of doses before the patient can say that they are truly better. In other situations the treatment will offer some release from a chronic condition, for which patients experience different symptoms with different intensities. As a result of our inherent variation, we do not respond to treatments in the same way and it is necessary to conduct clinical trials with a statistical end point to get an idea as to how well the treatment has worked and how well it will work in the general population.

What is statistics in the context of clinical trials?

Statistics are used to analyze the data from a clinical trial, and to test, or prove, the study hypothesis and confirm the primary objectives of the study. This is dependent on the phase of the study. In a Phase I study, the key information required is how much of the drug becomes available in the body. Drug concentration levels for the parent compound and its metabolites in the subject's plasma are sampled after the subject has ingested the drug by whatever administration route chosen (oral, intravenously (iv), intramuscularly (im). These samples are analyzed by the study pharmacokineticist or statistician to calculate key pharmacokinetic parameters: Cmax (maximum plasma concentration), tMax (time to maximum plasma concentration), AUC (area under the concentration-time curve), tHalf (elimination half-life). These parameters help to show how long the drug remains in the body, the level of maximum concentration and how much of the drug becomes available to the subject, see illustration below. Urine samples can also be collected and urine pharmacokinetic parameters calculated which relate to the elimination of the drug: Ae (0-t), Fe, CLr. (See Glossary.)

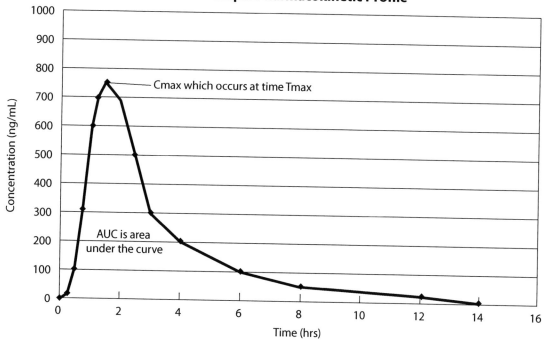

Example Pharmacokinetic Profile

Pharmacokinetics (Greek: 'pharmacon' = drug + 'kinetikos' = to put in motion) is the study of time dependency of a drug's action. The pharmacokinetic parameters are analyzed to confirm whether a new formulation is the same as an existing formulation (bioequivalent) by confirming that the Cmax and AUC of the new formulation are within certain pre-defined limits of the old formulation. Other analyses might show that increased doses are dose proportional, something that most clinicians prefer to see, or that there is no food effect (it doesn't matter if we take our medicine before or after a hearty meal), or that a modified release formulation has the same bioavailability (i.e., the fraction of a dose of an unchanged drug that reaches the systemic circulation) as an immediate release formulation with the same dose by analyzing the AUC. The analysis will take account of the study design; cross-over where subjects have received each of the treatments according to a randomized schedule, dose ascending where a new group of subjects receives the next dose. In addition to the results of analyzed data, there will be summary statistics relating to the other data recorded in the study. These will include descriptive summaries of the vital signs data at each time point and the number of subjects experiencing each adverse event and the severity.

Both Phase II and Phase III trials are designed to look more closely at the efficacy of the drug and also to monitor the safety. Phase II will also be used to select suitable doses. By the time the treatment is being used in Phase III studies there should be considerable information available from the early phase studies if it is a new drug or from published data if it is a new formulation of a known drug. For these trials, statistics are used to test the hypothesis defined in the protocol; the new treatment is better than the known treatment (superiority), or no worse than the known treatment (non-inferiority).

The hypothesis is set using existing knowledge of the drug or its mechanism and is quite specific in identifying potential differences that might be found. This information is used to calculate the number of subjects/patients needed for the study. At the end of the trial, the data are summarized and analyzed following the statistical analysis plan (SAP) or protocol which details how the data are to be summarized and analyzed. A study may have a primary variable such as a pain score or blood pressure, but the endpoint on which the analysis will be based is often a summary measure such as the average pain in the last week of taking medication, or the change in blood pressure from baseline. There is some scope to change the analysis plan before 'database lock' and subsequent unblinding of the data, but all changes need to be fully documented and, if necessary, a protocol amendment will need to be issued to detail the change and provide justification if the changes affect the primary endpoint. Generally, all of the data are listed and most of the data are summarized using descriptive statistics and a small number of endpoints identified for analysis. These endpoints are usually described as primary and secondary endpoints. The analysis used for the study will depend on the type of data that is recorded.

Why is statistics needed?

Statistics is needed in clinical trials to ensure that an appropriate number of subjects are recruited to the trial in order to have an acceptable chance of determining whether the new treatment works. It helps provide perspective on what the key outcomes from the study are. This is important because it is easy to get carried away and to record any number of variables because they might be of use and to analyze them. One of the problems caused by over-analysis of data is multiplicity, where the more analyses that are done, the greater the chance of finding something that is significant. Traditionally, most statistical tests are conducted at the 5% level, so that for every 20 analyses there will be one significant analysis.

Statistics is needed [for] confirming that the new treatment works

Statistical analysis of the data confirms or rejects the initial hypothesis. A quick glance at the mean value for two treatments may suggest that there is a very large difference, but the true extent of this difference will only be known once the data are analyzed. There may be quite a bit of variability which when taken into account shows that the apparent treatment difference doesn't exist. It may also be that there were too few subjects in the trial, which also results in failure to demonstrate a significant treatment difference. It is the role of statistics to quantify the likelihood that differences observed in the trial sample actually exist in the underlying population in the presence of variability.

Once the endpoints of the study have been defined, the sample size for the study can be estimated and the study design agreed upon. Most efficacy trials are conducted as parallel group designs where the subjects received one of the treatments according to a randomization schedule. Cross-over trials in which the subjects receive both or all of the treatments can be used and are often thought to be better because the subjects are acting as their own controls. However, they have their limitations because they can only be used successfully in chronic stable conditions for which there is a short treatment period. Many of the regulatory guidelines relating to the conduct of clinical trials in chronic conditions recommend long treatment periods (12 weeks or more) so that parallel group trials are more suitable. The study objectives must be clearly stated; will the new treatment definitely be better than the current gold standard, or is it more likely to show evidence that it has similar efficacy (equivalence) or that it is no worse. The FDA strongly encourages companies to discuss their clinical development plans with them and offers advice on the trial design and analysis. The documentation of the intended analysis in the protocol and statistical analysis plan ensures that the data are not trawled through to find a significant p-value for some obscure measurement. This follows the principles laid out by the International Conference on Harmonisation (ICH) and the CONSORT guidelines for publication ('Consolidated Standards of Reporting Trials' encompasses various initiatives to reduce problems from inadequate reporting of randomized controlled trials). Companies submitting regulatory dossiers to the FDA also submit the clinical trial data that is put into a standard format, so that the analysis can be replicated if the statistical assessor wishes. Dependent on the analysis and the assumptions made, the assessor may produce different results, which could impact on the submission. It is therefore essential that the intended analysis model is documented in the SAP and that the SAP is included with the dossier.

> The FDA strongly encourages companies to discuss their clinical development plans with them and offers advice on the trial design and analysis.

The future – trials are asking more questions

In the past, the clinical development plan would have included a number of small Phase I trials in which specific study objectives would have been investigated. These trials generally had a maximum of 40 subjects irrespective of the trial design, a cross-over bioequivalence or fed fasting study would have had about 24 completing subjects and a dose proportionality study would have had two subjects receiving placebo and six subjects receiving active drug for each of the, say, 5 dose levels under investigation. The trials were often run sequentially, so that the preliminary results were known before the next trial commenced, although some of the later trials may have been run in parallel. The process took time, which prolonged the time before the clinical stages of the product developmental plan could progress.

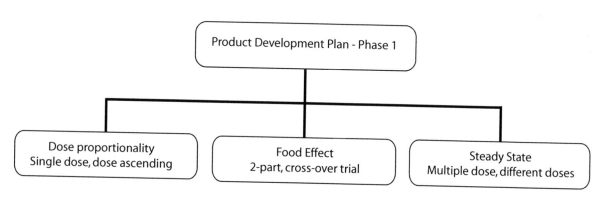

To speed a new product to market, drug developers prefer to speed up the clinical development and 'fast-track' the product for regulatory submission. This means in Phase I, a clinical trial may include a number of objectives to be investigated, and the trial may involve many more subjects. (See box, next page).

Companies are often interested in adaptive trial designs in which the sample size can be adjusted after a planned interim review. These adjustments can be done without losing the overall significance level of the trial. Recent developments in adaptive design mean that it is possible to make other changes during the course of a study such

Phase I study

An example of a Phase I study with an extended design is one in which the trial has two parts:

- ✦ Part 1, single dose and
- ✦ Part 2, steady state.

Part 1 will investigate the dose proportionality of the product by looking at the pharmacokinetic and pharmacodynamic properties of a single dose of the investigational product at increasing dose levels given to different groups of subjects. A small number of subjects in each dose group will also receive placebo. There will be a break between dosing at each dose level to allow time for the safety data (adverse events, lab data, ECGs) to be reviewed and a discussion taken on whether the next group of subjects should be dosed with the next dose level.

Part 2 will look specifically at questions relating to steady state such as the time taken to achieve steady state and the pharmacokinetic parameters associated with steady state, each group of subjects will receive one of the four dose levels under investigation. In addition to this, the study will look at the effects of food and gender, where subjects in one of the groups in Part 1 of the study will also take a single dose of the product after a high fat breakfast to investigate the effects of food, and one of the groups in the second part of the study will include an equal number of male and female subjects to see if there are any differences between male and female subjects on the pharmacokinetics of the product.

Although the study is complex and will take some time to complete as well as allowing for the safety review after each dose level during the single dose part of the study, there will be time saved by the company in terms of the time needed for protocol development, Phase I unit space, and ethics submissions and time before the results for objectives are obtained. For the statisticians and programmers responsible for summarizing and analyzing the data, there are a number of standard listings that should be produced whatever the size of the study, and although there will be some additional tables relating to the specific analyses that are to be conducted, they will have to produce fewer tables than if each question had been raised in a separate study as in the past. However, it is very important that all of the analyses that are required to answer questions raised by the protocol are fully documented in the SAP to ensure that they are conducted.

as the primary endpoint, primary analysis, or the planned treatment difference. These designs are being used to combine Phase II studies with larger Phase III studies. Such an approach provides greater efficiency for the developmental process.

Brief overview of the statistician's advisory and operational role on trials

Statisticians should be involved with every process of the clinical trial, although they will often have little involvement with the trial as it is ongoing, they should be aware of the issues that may arise during the course of the trial.

Protocol development

During protocol development, the statistician should be involved in deciding which study specific variables will be recorded in addition to standard data. These may also include biological markers that give an indication that the correct mode of action has been achieved.

They should help to define the study endpoints; whether variables will be summarized to create endpoints, or certain time points should be used. There should be input into the protocol, often writing the statistical analysis section to provide some detail on how the data will be summarized and analyzed and to identify the hypothesis for the study.

Sometimes it is necessary to discuss the clinical trial with the Regulatory Authorities (FDA in particular) and it is useful for the study statistician to attend to discuss specific statistical issues that may arise. For some therapeutic areas there are guidance notes on the trial design or the study duration that is expected for a study, and it is essential that this guidance is followed. Sample size calculations will be needed to see how many subjects are required for the study, these will differ dependent on the study endpoints and the assumptions made for the hypothesis. It is often necessary to review published literature to identify suitable measures from studies of a similar design.

Randomization

The statistician should be responsible for ensuring that the subjects are randomized to the study drugs in an appropriate manner. The process for randomization is dependent on the company conducting the trial, some companies use specific clinical trials software that links the randomization schedule with the drug packaging and others will rely on Statisticians to provide the schedule. For many Phase I studies the trial is open (i.e. not blinded) and the randomization schedule can be included in the CRF, in most cases when the study is blinded the subject is given a separate randomization number once they have fulfilled the study criteria. Sometimes a centralized randomization system may be used, but the Statistician will be responsible for reviewing blinded schedules.

Database

Although the statistician will not be responsible for annotating the CRF or creating the study database, they should be included in the review process to ensure that suitable variable names have been used and that there is consistency throughout the CRF.

SAP preparation

To ensure that the data are analyzed as planned, it is necessary to write a statistical analysis plan that should provide sufficient detail for another statistician or programmer to be able to write programs to summarize and analyze the data as required for the study. The SAP can be included as part of the protocol, but often it is a separate document which will include examples of code detailing how the analysis will be conducted or specific instructions on how data will be derived. The SAP will include mock-ups of listings and tables that will give a visual impression of how the data will be presented.

Analysis and summary of data

As the data are still being collected, the statistician and statistical programmers prepare SAS® (or other software) code to produce the analysis, tables and listings using either dummy data or study data (when it is possible to maintain the blind data, so as not to reveal treatment allocation codes). As a result of this 'blind' review, it may be necessary to recommend an alternative analysis from that documented in the protocol and SAP. All changes to the way in which the data are analyzed will need to be documented in the study report. If there are dramatic changes to the way in which the data are to be analyzed (particularly to the primary endpoint), it is necessary to issue a protocol amendment.

Once the study data are available for analysis (this will either be on study completion, or part way through if it is a planned interim analysis), the statistician needs to be able to provide summary tables, listings and analysis as quickly as possible. The ability to prepare programs in advance often using standard programs means that the tables and listings can be produced almost immediately once the randomization schedule has been released.

Reporting

Clinical Study Report: Previously, statisticians were responsible for writing a statistical report that documented the methods and results of the data analysis. This documentation was then used to contribute towards the Clinical Study Report (CSR). However, by creating an independent statistical report, additional time is added to the reporting process when most of the time the contents of the statistical report is rewritten to be put into the appropriate sections of the CSR. Many companies now follow an integrated approach where the results from the statistical analysis are written directly into the CSR with the statistician working very closely with the medical writer to ensure that the correct information is reported.

Publication: The results from all clinical studies, whether positive or negative, should be reported. The statistician is therefore involved in the preparation of manuscripts to report the results. Sometimes the results are reported in a poster at a relevant conference and statistical input is required to ensure the information is presented appropriately.

Regulatory submission: Although the statistician is not responsible for the submission of a regulatory dossier, he or she should be aware of the information that has been provided. Statisticians often pool the safety and efficacy results from the clinical trials to provide an integrated summary of safety and efficacy (ISSE) for the dossier. When questions come back from the regulatory agencies, the statisticians are often involved in answering them.

Summary and conclusion

In summary, the statistician is a core member of the clinical trial project team bringing valuable expertise to the design, mechanism of collection and interpretation of data. Appropriate input at the various key stages described above will enhance the quality of the trial and may also streamline the time taken to conduct the trial by the judicious prospective selection of the key data needed. Use your statistician wisely and ensure their full integration within the clinical project team.

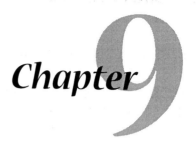

Chapter 9

The clinical trial process: what is data management?

Ms. Lisa Nash, GlaxoSmithKline

Data management, in essence, is the capture, validation and preparation of accurate clinical trial data for statistical analysis.

Introduction

Due to the diversity of the responsibilities within the data management umbrella, a clear and crisp definition is difficult to articulate, but here goes…

Data Management in essence, is the capture, validation and preparation of accurate clinical trial data for statistical analysis. Good data management requires maintaining the integrity of the data throughout each of the processes to which it is subjected.

Hopefully the information provided in this chapter will give you a clearer picture of the ever- evolving role of the data manager in the clinical trials process.

What is the data management environment like?

Data management is subjected to the same rigorous regulations, laws and guidelines, as the whole clinical trial process. Data management, as part of the sponsor's function has an obligation to protect the safety, dignity and well being of clinical trial subjects as well as maintaining confidentiality of patient data. As a result, it is critical for data managers to be conversant with the current guidances in the form of International Conference on Harmonisation (ICH) Good Clinical Practices (GCP), (which provides a framework for clinical trials in the EU, US and Japan). Managers must also understand the latest regulations applicable to the intended markets, e.g., the Code of Federal Regulations provided by the US Food and Drug Administration (FDA).

ICH GCP lays out guidance on quality control and assurance, data handling, record keeping and essential documents for clinical trial conduct.

As mentioned in more detail in the chapters on regulatory and ethical issues, ICH GCP describes the sponsors' responsibilities when 'designing, conducting, recording and reporting trials that involve the participation of human subjects.' For Data Management, ICH GCP lays out guidance on quality control and assurance, data handling, record keeping and essential documents for clinical trial conduct. It is, however, important for Data Managers to be aware of the wider responsibilities of the Investigator and Sponsor detailed in these guidelines, so they may highlight compliance risks as data is received.

The FDA's Title 21 CFR part 11 'sets forth the criteria under which the agency considers electronic records, electronic signatures and handwritten signatures executed to electronic records to be trustworthy, reliable and generally equivalent to paper records and handwritten signatures executed on paper'. In essence it describes the necessary considerations that need to be in place to ensure the accuracy and integrity of the electronic data at every step of the clinical trial process, from record creation, to modification, maintenance, retrieval and transmission.

Data Managers also need to be aware of the Clinical Trials Directive in the EU, which takes the guidance provided by ICH GCP and formalizes it within a legal framework. Our intention is not to provide a detailed list of applicable regulations here, as the regulations are constantly updated and quickly become obsolete. Please see the further reading section at the end of this chapter for useful links on this.

Brief overview of data management in clinical trials

Data management activities can be simplified and broken down into the following steps (also illustrated on the next page):

- ✦ Data capture
- ✦ Date entry*
- ✦ Data validation (including Serious Adverse Event, (SAE), reconciliation, coding and reconciliation of external data)
- ✦ Data integration (combining data from sources other than the case report form)
- ✦ Database lock (finalization or closure of the database)

* For studies using the paper process for collecting data

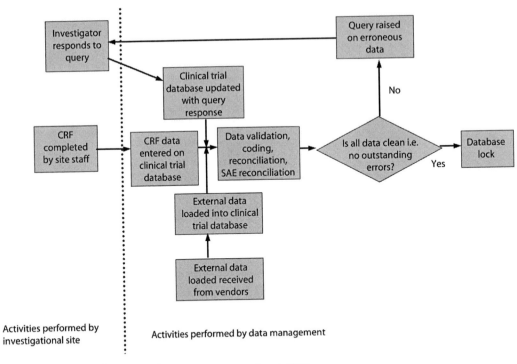

Figure 1: An example of a paper data management process.

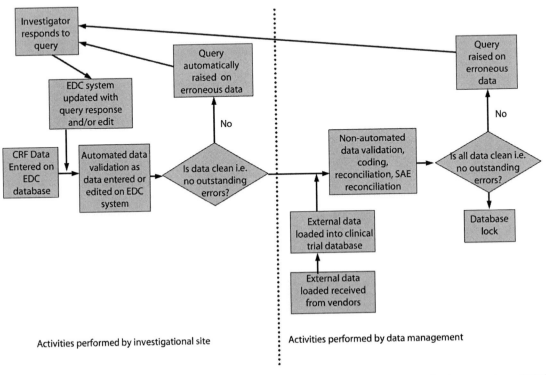

Figure 2: An example of an electronic data management process , with electronic data capture (EDC).

Data capture:

The scope of the data management function varies between organizations. Generally, the data management function is responsible for the data capture methodology implemented on a trial. Data may be gathered from investigational sites by paper means or by an electronic means. The paper or electronic document used to collect the data is commonly referred to as a case report form (CRF) - see examples below and on next page. Well-considered CRF design can dramatically improve the quality of the data collected from the investigational site ensuring the appropriate information is captured and reducing data cleaning resources later in the data management process. Data management groups often have a separate specialist CRF design functions dedicated to the design of paper CRFs or the building of electronic CRFs. (See also the chapter on technology in clinical trials).

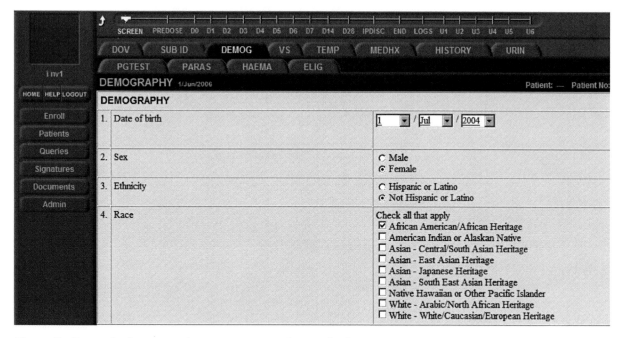

Figure 3: Example demography screen on an electronic data management system.

Example of a paper demography page

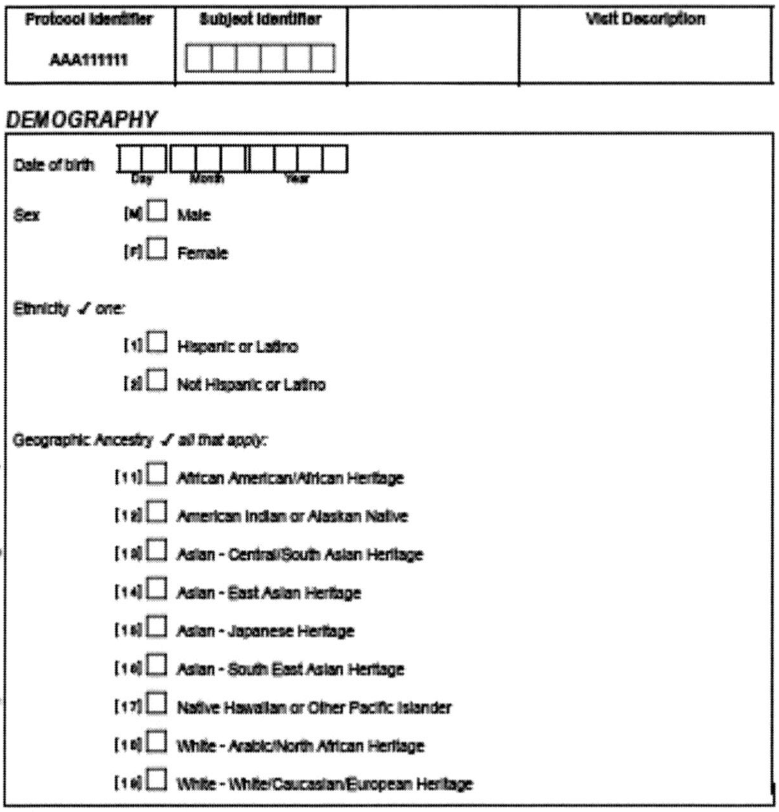

Protocol Identifier	Subject Identifier		Visit Description
AAA111111			

DEMOGRAPHY

Date of birth (Day / Month / Year)

Sex
[M] ☐ Male
[F] ☐ Female

Ethnicity ✓ *one:*
[1] ☐ Hispanic or Latino
[2] ☐ Not Hispanic or Latino

Geographic Ancestry ✓ *all that apply:*
[11] ☐ African American/African Heritage
[12] ☐ American Indian or Alaskan Native
[13] ☐ Asian - Central/South Asian Heritage
[14] ☐ Asian - East Asian Heritage
[15] ☐ Asian - Japanese Heritage
[16] ☐ Asian - South East Asian Heritage
[17] ☐ Native Hawaiian or Other Pacific Islander
[18] ☐ White - Arabic/North African Heritage
[19] ☐ White - White/Caucasian/European Heritage

Figure 4: Example of a paper demography page.

Data Entry:

Once completed at site the paper CRF will have the data verified against the source data (e.g. patient notes) by the monitor in a process known as source document verification. The CRF is then sent to the sponsor or contract house for data entry. This is where the data is entered into the clinical trial database. To ensure the accuracy of this data transcription step double data entry is commonly used. This double-entry of data from the same CRF, by two separate data entry clerks permits a real-time comparison as the data is entered by the second clerk. The system highlights any discrepancies between the two sets of data entered by the clerks during entry. An alternative comparison method can be used whereby a separate compare program is run that outputs errors for correction separately. Alternatively, a company may use a single entry method and a manual quality control process. These days, there are fewer trials where the data is collected via paper CRFs, so data entry at the sponsor or contract house site is being reduced. Electronic data capture (EDC) methodologies shift this process to the investigational sites. This can create different challenges for the data management department at the sponsor and investigational site.

Data validation:

Data validation is the process of ensuring that the data is accurate, and truly reflects what happened to a particular subject during his or her inclusion in the clinical trial. Validation is a key activity throughout the life of the trial and is the responsibility of all those involved in the trial. This includes the creator of the initial clinical trial data, i.e. the investigator, and extends through to every individual (monitors, data managers, statisticians, etc …). It is a critical aspect of every process that handles the data, right through to the final clinical report and submission.

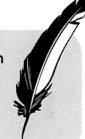

Data validation is becoming increasingly automated.

Data validation from a data management perspective commences once the data is received from the investigator. Once clinical trial data is entered into the clinical trial database, either by the trial site staff on an EDC system, or by the data entry function, data management staff are able to view the data and commence the data validation steps. Data validation is, in essence, the review of the data to check its accuracy and consistency in relation to the clinical trial. Data validation is becoming increasingly automated, using programmatic checks or automatic checks within the EDC system as the data is entered. EDC systems contain this checking and query management functionality as part of the package. These systems are often referred to as electronic data management (EDM) systems. Manual checking does however still have a place in the data validation process.

Accuracy and consistency checks run on clinical trial data

Examples of accuracy checks include

- ✦ checking laboratory data results are compatible with life
- ✦ ensuring dates are consistent with participation in the clinical trial
- ✦ identifying protocol violators
- ✦ highlighting missing data
- ✦ checking values are within expected ranges for that population.

Consistency checks are generally more complex. For example, investigational product compliance records may indicate that a subject stopped study medication due to an adverse experience. The check would then look for an adverse experience consistent with the stopping date of the investigational product. Consistency checks may involve checking data from different sources, for example, the investigational site and a third party vendor, such as an ECG vendor.

> [T]he number of validation checks run over the data … has been known to pass the thousand mark!

Given the complexity and detail of the data collected for clinical trials the number of validation checks run over the data is often in the hundreds and has been known to pass the thousand mark! Once the potential errors have been highlighted, data queries are generated and sent to the investigational sites. In an ideal world the data queries would highlight a data entry error, which is easily resolved by the entry of the correct value. More often than not the query highlights a genuine error, e.g. out of range lab value due to sample problems. Depending on the response to the data query raised, this may highlight wider issues that data management should make a study team aware of. These issues might include problems such as an investigational site consistently not following the protocol, by not performing certain protocol-defined tests, or not following sample handling procedures. If data entry and validation are performed in-stream, e.g. data is handled on an ongoing basis, then corrective measures can be taken while the trial is still active.

Serious adverse events:

Serious adverse events (SAEs)[1], are frequently collected and 'databased' by the sponsor's pharmacovigilence group, using a specifically designed safety database to expedite regulatory reporting of investigation product related events. Often the same information is gathered within the CRF or eCRF data that is received by data management. When this is the case, a reconciliation step needs to occur to ensure that the data within the clinical trial database and safety database concur. Pharmacovigilance departments often make contact with the investigator to request the additional data to clarify the case. These changes are not always updated by the investigator in the CRF, leading to discrepancies being identified when the SAE reconciliation step is performed between the two databases. In cases where discrepancies are identified queries need to be raised for the investigational site to clarify the data. As such, SAE reconciliation activities are performed during the data validation phase of a trial, prior to database lock.

Editing of the clinical trial data:

The responses to data queries frequently result in the need to edit the data. For example, the initial data entry included a transcription error, or additional information came to light, changing the original response. Where a paper CRF has been used to collect trial data the edits will need to be made to the clinical trial database. These will be performed by the data management group. For electronic CRFs, depending on the set up of the system, the edits will either be performed by the investigational site or by the data management group. For any clinical trial database or system the maintenance of an accurate audit trail from the creation of the record through each subsequent update made to that record is important. It should be possible to identify which system user made the edit, the date it was made, what the original value was and to be able to trace the reason for the edit.

---

1 According to the US FDA, an adverse event is any undesirable experience associated with the use of a medical product in a patient. The event is 'serious' and should be reported when the patient outcome is: Death, life-threatening, hospitalization required, disability, congenital anomaly (suspicions that exposure to a medical product prior to conception or during pregnancy resulted in an adverse outcome in the child), requires intervention to prevent permanent impairment or damage.

Coding of medical terms and medications:

Coding is the process by which certain terms collected within the clinical trial data are databased and have a numeric, alphabetic or alphanumeric code assigned to them. As recently as 15 years ago this was primarily a manual process where codes or phrases from a medical terminology were entered into a database, as databases were unable to hold long strings of text. Technology has become increasingly powerful and this is not an issue these days. The need for coding is now mainly to support the provision of data to regulatory authorities in a variety of formats for a variety of purposes. As such, standard medical terminologies have been developed. The International Conference for Harmonisation (ICH) developed the Medical Dictionary for Regulatory Activities (MedDRA), which is owned by the International Federation of Pharmaceutical Manufacturers and Associations (IFPMA). This is described on the MedDRA website (www.meddramsso.com) as, 'a pragmatic, medically valid terminology with an emphasis on ease of use for data entry, retrieval, analysis, and display, as well as a suitable balance between sensitivity and specificity within the regulatory environment.'

> The MedDRA dictionary is arranged in a five level hierarchy:
>
> LLT   Lower Level Term
>
> PT   Preferred Term
>
> HLT   High Level Term
>
> HLGT   High Level Group Term
>
> SOC   System Organ Class

These levels are arranged with the most specific, LLT at the top of this list, descending to the most general level, SOC. The LLTs are the most specific level of the terminology and reflect "common usage". MedDRA is updated and new releases are available every 6 months, this allows the inclusion of new terms and associations to be amended.

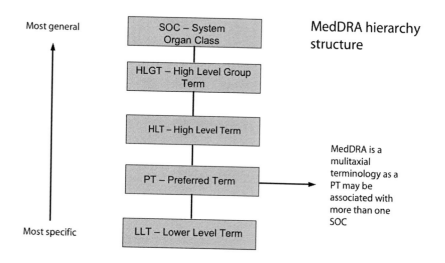

Figure 5: An example of the MedDRA hierarchy as demonstrated with a PT of headache.

Each of the terms listed below is grouped under the same Preferred Term of 'Headache', so during data analysis all of these terms will be group together as they are medically related.

SOC: Nervous system disorder

HLGT: Headaches

HLT: Headaches NEC

PT : Headache

LLTs:

- Cephalgia
- Forehead headache
- Fullness head
- Head fullness
- Head pain
- Head pressure
- Head throbbing
- Headache
- Headache (except migraine) aggravated
- Headache dull
- Headache fullness
- Headache NOS

- Headache NOS aggravated
- Headache occurring
- Headache temporal
- Headache transient
- Nocturnal headache
- Pain head
- Pounding in head
- Temporal headache
- Headache aggravated
- Frontal headache
- Occipital headache
- Parietal headache

- Premenstrual headache
- Headache unilateral
- Drug-induced headache
- Frequent headaches
- Chronic headaches
- Headache (excl. migraine) aggravated
- Throbbing headache
- Intermittent headache
- Retroauricular pain
- Headache recurrent

What data types are coded? Typically adverse events and medical procedures are coded, although some organizations also code medical histories. For example, adverse events are collected for patients during their participation in a clinical trial. By coding the data it is possible to analyze the number of instances of medical events. This also enables consistency in reviewing the data. For example, using MedDRA, headache, sore head, cephalgia would be grouped together under the same PT because they have the same essential medical meaning. This mechanism also allows the consistent interpretation of data in different languages.

MedDRA has been specifically designed to be applicable to all phases of development including post marketing activities, excluding animal toxicology. It covers terms relating to adverse events (diagnoses as well as signs and symptoms), medical procedures, a variety of investigations and social circumstances. As this has been adopted by ICH this makes review of the coded data easier for the regulatory authorities, as standard groupings are applied across the pharmaceutical industry.

> MedDRA has been specifically designed to be applicable to all phases of development including post marketing activities.

Data integration:

The clinical trial process is increasingly being influenced by the evolution of technology designed to improve the quality of patient care. For example digital outputs from ECG machines allow real-time transmission of cardiology data via the world wide web to a cardiologist for review, on the far side of the globe. It is commonplace for laboratory data to be received electronically from central labs within many organizations. A wide range of scan data is also now available electronically from specialist vendors. With the increase in the variety of sources from which electronic clinical data may be received, the data manager is faced with the challenge of integrating all these electronic data with the clinical trial database to provide a consolidated batch of data for statistical analysis. The magnitude of the challenge presented by this will be dependent on the process and system set up within the individual organization.

Patient reported outcomes:

Patient reported outcomes are becoming more and more common in trials. These may monitor a variety of things from moods, to rash coverage to bowel movements, depending on the indication of the trial. Many psychiatric trials use validated rating scales for subjects to identify how they are feeling on a frequent basis. The difficulty for the data manager is ensuring the cleanliness of the data. Paper reported outcomes may be collected in paper diaries or electronic diaries, with either route there is a delay in the receipt of the data at data management ranging from a few days to weeks, making it impossible to query missing data on the condition of a subject on a specific date. There are many operational challenges when collecting patient reported outcomes relating to patient compliance. Many electronic vendors can identify if subjects are completing the information as they should, e.g. on a daily basis or in all in one go just prior to their visit to the investigator. This is a huge benefit to demonstrating reliability of the data collected. Ensuring subjects transmit electronic data on regular basis can also prove tricky making it difficult for data management to highlight possible issues in-stream.

If an electronic diary is being used from an external vendor, this is another data stream that will need to be integrated with the clinical trial data for reporting. Paper data may be entered directly into the clinical trial database.

Database lock:

Once the all the data is received and deemed fully 'cleaned', so there are no unresolved queries at the clinical trial site, and so all reconciliations are resolved and all medical terms are coded, the data is ready for statistical analysis. To ensure that no further changes to the data can be made the database is 'locked' or 'frozen.' Here all access is revoked, although a number of organizations permit read-only access in case questions arise during the analysis and reporting process. Making data available for review to the statisticians prior to database lock facilitates early issue resolution and reduces the incidence of issues requiring site clarification and potential data changes post database lock.

Summary and conclusion

The benefits of data management:

A well-nurtured clinical data management department has a positive impact on the whole clinical trial process. Through investment in building therapeutic expertise, technical and project management skills, data managers can add value at all steps of the trial from protocol design to reporting. The clinical data management department can review protocols and provide input to sections of the protocol, clarifying areas that were problematic in other studies. Also the data manager can contribute to therapeutic discussions and sometimes highlight aspects or risks encountered in similar studies, not yet considered by the team. Support can also be provided at investigator and monitor meetings to provide training on CRF completion and query processes, providing detailed expectations to attendees and highlight common pitfalls. This helps improve the quality of the data provided by the investigator to the sponsor. During the time that a trial is active, data management can support the team in decision-making by providing data for review to the agreed quality (i.e. in-stream unvalidated data, or clean data) as well as contributing to discussions based on their experience or knowledge.

The analysis and reporting process is an important area and one where data managers must have a good understanding. Data management can keep the reporting team informed of population details and highlight if expected targets will not be met and the reasons provided within the data received. Having a good understanding of the reporting plan allows data management to focus data cleaning and quality assurance activities to the most critical data, ensuring the data is fit for purpose without excessively large effort being spent on less important data.

Data management departments play a key role with study teams as they can influence the quality of the study through an enhanced understanding of the data they are handling, and through a better understanding of what the teams are trying to achieve through the protocol. Having direct contact with investigational sites and monitors can provide swift and focused data issue resolution by highlighting common problems. Depending on the flexibility of systems and processes within the organization, the data management function may have a choice of systems that can be used for the trial, so getting the data manager involved early allows them to select the most robust data capture solution to meet the demands of the study.

In conclusion, data management is a dynamic field. With the spiraling costs of research and development required to get products to market, the pressure to reduce time from discovery to product launch increases. This ensures that data management departments are constantly seeking ways to speed up data collection, cleaning and provision of the data for reporting. The importance of data being cleaned and available in-stream is increasing rapidly to expedite safety reviews so companies can make decisions around discontinuing compound investment at earlier stages within trials.

Recommended reading

For those interested in learning more about data management in clinical trials, you may wish to review the following:

Book:

*   Clinical Data Management by Richard Rondel, Sheila Varley and Colin Webb, published by Wiley.

Associations:

*   Association for Clinical Data Management (ACDM) website: www.acdm.org.uk
*   Society for Clinical Data Management (SCDM) website: www.scdm.org

Other useful links:

*   MedDRA website: www.meddramsso.com
*   CFR21 Index can be found on the FDA website: http://www.fda.gov
*   EU Clinical trials directive http://www.eortc.be/Services/Doc/clinical-EU-directive-04-April-01.pdf
*   ICH GCP: http://www.emea.europa.eu/pdfs/human/ich/013595en.pdf

Chapter 10

The clinical trials process: technology in clinical trials

Bill Byrom, VP Product Management,
ClinPhone plc, Nottingham, UK

David Stein VP Product Management,
ClinPhone Inc, Princeton, NJ, USA

Technology application promises to simplify processes and logistics in the management of complex and geographically diverse clinical trials.

Introduction

Over the past two decades, clinical trials have become larger and more complex and this trend is continuing. In addition, clinical trials have become increasingly global. Multinational studies are commonplace and conducted in a growing list of countries, all of which provide important access to patient populations and pre-approval exposure within potentially important markets.

In addition, the integrity and precision of data collected is under increased scrutiny and quality expectations. Pharmaceutical sponsors are subject to greater examination of safety issues and regulators demand increased information on a new drug's safety profile both pre- and post-approval. For example, it is now a formal requirement to conduct a thorough electrocardiogram (ECG) study on every new drug being developed, the result of which may lead to additional ECG monitoring and analysis throughout the entire development program.

> it is now a formal requirement to conduct a thorough elec-trocardiogram (ECG) study on every new drug being developed.

It is not surprising that many analysts report spiraling costs of clinical research, and as a consequence sponsors seek to accelerate development programs in order to achieve return on their investment sooner and with longer patent protection remaining.

Technology plays a major role in meeting these challenges in today's clinical trials. Technology application promises to simplify processes and logistics in the management of complex and geographically diverse clinical trials. It also promises to improve the quality and integrity of data collected, and to accelerate the overall time taken to conduct studies.

In this chapter we examine the application and benefits of technologies that have become increasingly commonplace in today's clinical trials, namely:

✦ Central randomization and trial supply management solutions
✦ Electronic Data Capture (EDC) systems
✦ Electronic Patient Reported Outcomes (ePRO) solutions
✦ Clinical Trial Management Systems (CTMS).

Central randomization and trial supply management solutions

The acceleration of clinical research often means that studies must start with shorter lead times and less raw material and hence fewer supplies available. Moreover, the logistics of ensuring study sites remain appropriately stocked with study medication and managing expiry dates across multi-site, multinational studies is a significant management task.

How IVR/IWR trial supply management solutions work

Consider how a supermarket limits running out of stock of each item on their shelves, whilst minimizing the quantity of stock stored locally. Electronic Point Of Sales (EPOS) systems automate the re-ordering of stock by tracking inventories based upon sales recorded through the check out. IVR/IWR trial supply management solutions follow the same concept in tracking medication usage each time it is dispensed to a patient and using this information to automate re-stocking of sites.

Using IVR/IWR, drug supplies are not packaged in patient-numbered kits, but each dispensing unit of medication is assigned a unique numerical code. In a repeat dispensing study, for example, this means that a different pack is dispensed at each dispensing visit. This feature generates flexibility in the supplies: any pack at site can be assigned to any patient (within the appropriate treatment group); it is not necessary to store all packs potentially required by an individual patient up front; and packs earmarked for patients that subsequently withdraw can be allocated to other patients

Clinical trial supply management solutions reduce the quantity of medication required by an individual study by optimizing the supply chain and automatically directing supplies to depots and sites when they are needed. These solutions commonly use the telephone and web as the interface with the user and are often referred to as Interactive Voice Response (IVR) and Interactive Web Response (IWR).

Interactive Voice Response (IVR) systems

For those unfamiliar with IVR, these systems use the telephone as an interface between the end-user and a central computer. Voice files recorded in local language are played to relay messages, ask questions and present menu options. A typical Investigator menu might be:

1 randomize a new patient
2 re-dispense to an existing patient
3 identify withdrawal or completion of a patient
4 acknowledge arrival of a medication shipment
5 perform emergency code-break.

within the same treatment group. These features mean that the quantity of stock stored at each site can be minimized and the amount of medication wasted due to patient withdrawals and low patient recruitment can be limited, while maintaining the study blind.

Figure 1 illustrates simplistically how an IVR/IWR system operates to control medication allocation and maintain sufficient stock levels at site.

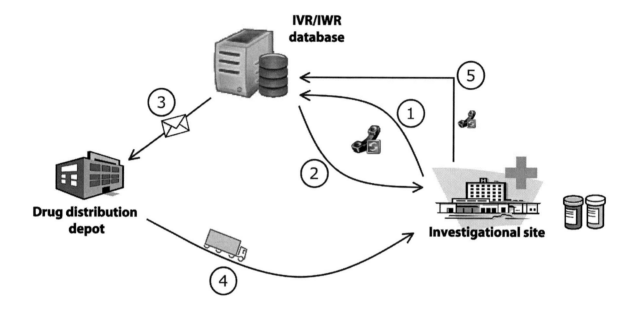

KEY

(1) Investigator makes a toll-free call to randomize a patient or dispense medication

(2) The system reports the medication pack number to be allocated, based upon the randomization schedule. This information is normally confirmed by an automated fax or email.

(3) When site stock levels fall to a pre-defined minimum level, the system generates a shipment request for a defined quantity of medication by fax or email to the distribution depot

(4) Medication is shipped to site

(5) The site acknowledges receipt of the medication shipment and the system updates the central database with the new packs available.

Figure 1: Automated supply chain management using IVR/IWR.

Central randomization and emergency code break

Importantly, in the process of managing medication dispensation and site inventories, IVR/IWR solutions also perform the randomization of subjects to treatments according to the method required by the protocol. Central randomization brings a number of benefits:

1. It eliminates the potential for errors in treatment assignment that may occur when sites are responsible for this activity.

2. It enables more complex randomization methods to be applied, such as when it is desirable to ensure treatment groups contain similar proportions of patients with certain characteristics that are believed to influence treatment response. An example may be in diabetes where body weight and baseline fasting blood glucose (or HbA1c) may influence the magnitude of treatment response. Common methods may include stratification and dynamic allocation methods such as minimization.

3. It provides a real-time picture of study recruitment performance enabling study teams to plan monitoring visits, determine contingencies when experiencing low recruitment, and close the study rapidly without significant over-recruitment.

4. Enables emergency code break using IVR. This removes the need to provide sites and sponsor personnel with code break envelopes, ensure on-call personnel are within easy reach of the envelopes, and eliminates any uncertainty regarding whether a code break envelope has been opened or tampered with.

Benefits of IVR/IWR randomization and trial supply management

1	Simplify the logistics of managing the clinical trial supply chain, particularly in multi-center, multinational studies.
2	Reduced drug wastage and overage.
3	Enable complex randomization methods to be applied that would be difficult or impossible using traditional site-based randomization methods.
4	Provide real-time enrolment and study progress reports for effective study management
5	Perform emergency code break by telephone from any location without the need for code break envelopes

Electronic Data Capture (EDC) solutions

Traditionally, clinical trials data recorded by the Investigator are recorded on paper Case Report Forms (CRFs). These forms contain fields for all the required measurements and recordings to be entered – for example a demographics form may contain fields for age, date of birth, gender, height, weight and race. Forms are presented in a book with specific forms used at different scheduled patient assessment visits based upon the requirements of the study (defined in the study Protocol). Although this is a simple approach, using paper records has a number of disadvantages including:

1. Data collected at site are only available to the Sponsor and Data Management team once collected at a monitoring visit. This may introduce a lag of 6-8 weeks in data being entered into the Sponsor's clinical data management system and the data cleaning and checking process commencing.

2. Data queries generated by the monitor, data manager or medical reviewer may be received by the study site some weeks after the data were collected, which may limit their ability to respond accurately.

> **EDC can provide enormous efficiency into the data collection and cleaning process required by clinical trials.**

3. Time from last patient last visit to database lock may be weeks because of the delay in receiving data and the delay in generating and resolving queries.

4. Data recorded on paper may be ambiguous or illegible.

5. Paper records for a complete clinical trial are high volume and may require subsequent micro-filming to ensure records can be retained in an archive for the required timeframe post-study.

6. Even when stored securely, paper records may be lost or damaged.

EDC solutions use electronic Case Report Forms (eCRFs) for sites to record their clinical assessment data. These typically use internet-connected PCs. By using a web-browser users are able to securely connect to the central EDC application to review and enter data.

EDC can provide enormous efficiency into the data collection and cleaning process required by clinical trials. Monitors and study directors can view site clinical assessment data as soon as it has been entered – often at, or shortly following, a patient visit. This facilitates rapid data review and feedback to the study site if data queries are found. EDC solutions contain functionality that enables monitors and data managers to raise queries against data points or forms completed, and for investigators to provide written responses to queries and make changes to data with the database retaining a full history of data changes and reasons for these.

This significantly accelerates the data cleaning process and ensures that queries are raised in a timely manner so that accurate responses can be made and quality, clean data achieved quickly. In addition to manual queries, EDC solutions can contain automated logic checks contained within the electronic forms so that immediate data queries can be raised as data are entered, such as flagging out-of-range values.

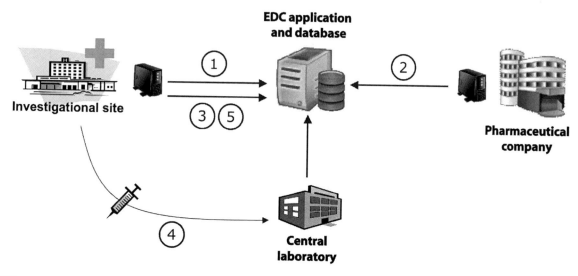

KEY

(1) Investigator enters clinical assessment data on-line using a web-connected PC.

(2) Sponsor personnel review data remotely and raise manual queries.

(3) Investigator responds to queries and makes changes to the data if appropriate.

(4) Investigator sends blood samples for analysis at the central laboratory. These data are issued electronically and automatically imported into the eCRFs.

(5) Investigator reviews and, if appropriate, comments on lab results.

Figure 2: Typical workflow when using an Electronic Data Capture System.

As illustrated in Figure 2, another efficiency of EDC arises from the ability to import data automatically from other sources. For example, the results of blood sample analyses conducted at a central laboratory can be securely transferred electronically and automatically uploaded into the appropriate eCRF for the Investigator to review and comment against. This efficiency applies to other sources of data – such as electronic patient diaries which can feed data in real time into the EDC solution enabling the investigator to review patient progress outside clinic visits. This prevents the requirement to re-enter data, and ensures that all data referring to the patient is able to be inspected and reviewed through a single application – the EDC system.

Although EDC enables clinical data to be reviewed and monitored remotely, using an EDC system does not mean that monitors are not required to attend sites for regular site visits. Source data verification (SDV) activities are still an important requirement, and these can only be conducted on site. Many EDC applications provide the means of recording these activities against the data verified. Ideally, the monitor is able to spend time at site conducting SDV and spending valuable time with site personnel, without the need to spend significant time reviewing the CRFs as this is performed in advance rather than conducted during the visit.

Benefits of EDC

1	Reduced time to database lock.
2	Faster query turnaround time and reduced volume of queries.
3	No requirement for in-house double data entry resource.
4	More efficient use of time at monitoring visits.
5	Efficient and simple site and study data archiving.

Electronic Patient Reported Outcomes (ePRO) solutions

Patient reported outcomes data are an important component of many clinical development programs. In some therapy areas where the effects of treatment are hard for a clinician to measure at clinic, symptom diaries maintained by the patient represent the most valuable data providing information on drug efficacy. Examples may include sleep diaries for insomnia treatments, diaries to record migraine symptoms or pain diaries in studies of pain relief therapy. In addition to this, patient reported data can provide valuable quality of life and secondary data that may influence the drug labeling claims.

Traditionally, patient reported outcomes (PRO) data have been collected using paper diaries supplied to the patient for home use. Since the turn of the millennium there has been a rapidly growing interest in the electronic collection of these data, and a growing weight of evidence indicating serious concerns and limitations with diary data collected on paper. Possibly the most interesting of these was published in the British Medical Journal in 2002[1] in which researchers supplied patients with a paper diary containing a hidden microchip which recorded when the diary was opened and closed. This enabled the researchers to identify whether diary entries were recorded at times scheduled by the protocol, or at other times – such as just prior to a clinic appointment. The study affirmed the fear that patient compliance with paper diary completion, although apparently high based upon the number of records entered, lacked integrity as many entries were recorded retrospectively – and some patients even completed their diary ahead of time! It's unlikely that you can remember what you had for dinner a week ago, and similarly this brings into question the accuracy and integrity of paper diary data which may be recorded many days after the event in question. In addition, because paper diaries are normally completed by patients in an unsupervised environment, this often results in significant data quality limitations as illustrated in figure 3.

> **Electronic patient diaries provide a way of improving data quality and demonstrating the timeliness of diary entries.**

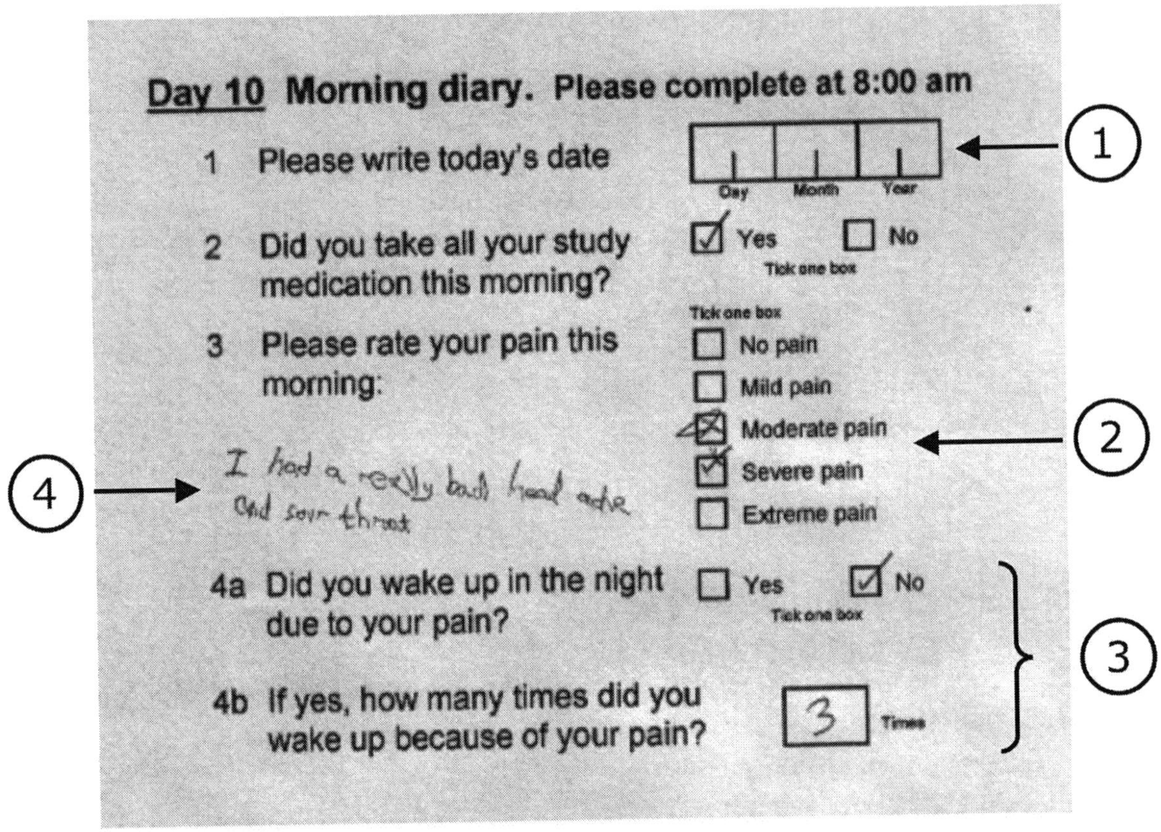

Day 10 Morning diary. Please complete at 8:00 am

1 Please write today's date — Day / Month / Year

2 Did you take all your study medication this morning? ☑ Yes ☐ No (Tick one box)

3 Please rate your pain this morning: (Tick one box)
☐ No pain
☐ Mild pain
☒ Moderate pain
☑ Severe pain
☐ Extreme pain

I had a really bad head ache and sore throat

4a Did you wake up in the night due to your pain? ☐ Yes ☑ No (Tick one box)

4b If yes, how many times did you wake up because of your pain? 3 Times

Figure 3: Example of data quality issues with a simple paper diary.

KEY

(1) Missing data.
(2) Ambiguous data.
(3) Conflicting data.
(4) Extraneous data.

Electronic patient diaries provide a way of improving data quality and demonstrating the timeliness of diary entries. Both these attributes are important when PRO data are included in a new drug application to a regulatory body. Commonly employed solutions include hand-held devices such as personal digital assistants and Interactive Voice Response systems, although the web has also been used in some clinical trials. In each case, the patient is able to enter data, which is received by a central study database either immediately (IVR, hand-held devices with wireless (mobile) transmission) or once the data are physically sent (such as when the device modem is connected to a telephone line (non-wireless hand-held devices)).

EPRO solutions can be configured to include logic checks that prohibit the entry of conflicting or ambiguous data, and can be made to record the time and date of entries, enabling researchers to measure and demonstrate the timeliness of diary recordings. Pre-defined time-windows can also prohibit entries from being made at improper times.

When using an ePRO solution, the choice of solution will depend upon the type of data collected, frequency of use, and capabilities of the patient population. In general, most solutions are simple enough to be used in most studies. Interactive Voice Response diaries have advantages in that no equipment needs to be supplied or maintained in the field – patients use their home telephones. Alternatively, hand-held devices have a greater ability to collect certain types of data – such as visual analogue scale recordings.

> [P]atient diary data is defined by regulators as part of the case history of the patient and is therefore the responsibility of the Investigator.

When employing an ePRO solution it is important to remember that patient diary data is defined by regulators as part of the case history of the patient and is therefore the responsibility of the Investigator. Unless the data are likely to lead to unblinding (for example, by revealing whether the patient is taking placebo or active drug) it is important that (as when using a paper diary) the study site has the ability to inspect the diary data and review it as part of their ongoing care for the patient.

Benefits of ePRO solutions

1	Ability to demonstrate and influence the timeliness of patient diary entries.
2	Improved data quality: reduced missing, conflicting, ambiguous, illegible and extraneous data.
3	Improved clinical monitoring of patients by access to patient reported data outside clinic visits, or automatic alerts generated by the ePRO solution.
4	Real-time diary compliance reporting, enabling encouragement to be given to patients who have ceased making diary entries.
5	No requirement for double-data entry of the PRO data.

Clinical Trial Management Systems (CTMS)

Clinical trials are complex to manage. There are numerous activities that need coordination and tracking from obtaining ethics approvals corresponding to each study site, to making appropriate and timely investigator payments. Many pharmaceutical companies use in-house-developed or commercially available Clinical Trial Management Systems to track and report the progress of all the clinical trials under their direction. These solutions enable trial directors to track the fine detail of all activities required by their clinical trial, and senior management to view higher level summary metrics on the progress of the entire development program of studies, or the complete portfolio of trials being conducted across all development programs.

CTMS' aim to manage the planning and track the performance of clinical trials. They have a number of functions and applications including:

1. Maintaining up-to-date contact information for key trial participants – such as key study site personnel, vendors and partners.

2. Tracking deadlines and milestones such as regulatory and ethics approvals.

3. Maintaining and producing monitoring reports for each Clinical Research Associate (CRA, (Monitor)) site visit.

4. Tracking and reporting patient screening, recruitment and completion metrics.

> CTMS are web-based systems allowing clinical program information to be shared with key stakeholders no matter where they are located geographically.

5. Managing the allocated study budget and determining and actioning investigator and vendor payments based upon study activities and progress performed.

6. Tracking drug shipments and site-based drug reconciliation activity.

7. Providing reports on all aspects of study progress and budget.

Many CTMS solutions have the ability to integrate with other systems used by the pharmaceutical company in the management of a clinical trial. For example, a CTMS may interface with the company's financial management system to enable payments authorized within the CTMS to be executed automatically. In addition, a CTMS may receive live study progress data from an EDC or IVR solution so that patient progress data are up-to-date rather than accurate to the last monitoring visit.

Many CTMS solutions have off-line functionality that enable the study monitor to input information via their laptop while at a site visit. This significantly increases the speed at which monitoring visit reports can be generated and accurate patient progress data maintained within the CTMS.

Increasingly, CTMS are web-based systems allowing clinical program information to be shared with key stakeholders no matter where they are located geographically. With the globalization of clinical trials, web-based systems have become increasingly important.

Benefits of CTMS

1	Tracking and reporting study planning progress against key milestones such as ethics and regulatory approvals.
2	Provision of accurate and comprehensive study progress information. This facilitates effective and timely management decisions, such as opening additional sites when recruitment is below target.
3	Management of the study budget and ensuring that investigator and vendor payments are made correctly and in timely manner.
4	Generating and maintaining monitoring reports.
5	Providing high-level management information across suites of studies for senior management.

Other technologies

In this chapter we have explored four key technologies routinely used in today's clinical trials. Of course, many existing and emerging technologies have a role to play in the effective conduct and implementation of our clinical development programs. For example, many studies use central reading and interpretation of complex clinical assessments such as ECGs and imaging. These require technology solutions to capture and transmit images and traces to a central repository where they can be accessed and interpreted by experts. In other clinical trials, medication is packaged in special medication compliance devices that are used to obtain an accurate picture of medication taking behavior, and how this influences health outcomes. In addition, most sponsors use pharmacovigilance systems to consolidate and analyze adverse events data and collect and manage the reporting of serious adverse events. There is much information available on these other technologies – simply walking the exhibition space at a large clinical trials conference will uncover many.

The future of technology in clinical trials

Technology solutions, such as those described above, are being used much more frequently in clinical trials. In many cases these solutions are used in isolation, while others require common data. This results in duplication of effort and reconciliation activities to ensure the accuracy and currency of each database. More frequently, clinical technology organizations and sponsor companies are employing integrated solutions whereby common data entered in a single solution are fed into other solutions requiring them. For example,

- ✦ IVR solutions may feed real-time patient progress data into a CTMS and dispensing data into an EDC solution;
- ✦ ePRO solutions may feed data directly into an EDC application;
- ✦ CTMS applications may interface directly with finance and billing applications;
- ✦ EDC applications may connect directly with automated medical coding solutions and pharmacovigilance systems.

In addition, data from all solutions may be consolidated to enable powerful far-reaching reporting of all aspects of a clinical trial's progress and data. The end result is efficient workflows, accurate data and elimination of duplicate activities and data reconciliation. This integrated environment is the next step in the effective use of technology in clinical trials.

References

1. Stone A. *et al.* (2002) Patient non-compliance with paper diaries. *British Medical Journal;* 324:1193-1194.

Chapter 11

The clinical trials process: medical writing

Ms. Fiona Swain, Swain Associates

Diplomacy is part of the
medical writer's job.

Introduction

The medical writer

What is the role of the medical writer?

As with all good scientific research, good documentation is essential to the clinical trial process. The medical writer plays a key role in the production of this documentation, particularly the final Clinical Study Report.

It's probably true to say that medical writing is an art. It takes a certain amount of skill to make complex concepts readily accessible to the reader. It is also true to say that not everyone relishes the task of writing, even if they have spent the last few months or years actively involved in the research. There is, therefore, a clear opportunity for a specialized writer to be involved and add value to the process.

Most pharmaceutical companies have a medical writing department or an outsourcing manager who employs freelance medical writers to fulfil this function. Medical writers mainly come from a scientific background and have a higher educational degree. New medical writers may enter the profession directly from education or indirectly from another branch of the pharmaceutical industry.

> **Medical communications is designed to create a suitable environment into which a medical product can be launched.**

The medical writer does not write in isolation, but is part of a team. Each document will have an authoring team who have to agree, not on only the general messages within each document, but also on the exact wording. This means that the medical writer interacts with a variety of people, each of whom has a different perspective. Diplomacy is therefore part of the medical writer's job. A good medical writer can facilitate the production of a document in a way that minimizes or removes the potential conflict and pain.

Another area in which medical writing has grown in importance is within the medical communications environment. Medical communications is designed to create a suitable environment into which a medical product can be launched by combining scientific and medical facts with core product marketing. A variety of media are used to communicate the right scientific messages arising from the trials of the product in a balanced and impartial way, drawing out strengths and addressing any potential limitations. This approach involves targeting a wide range of audiences and may encompass a number of disease areas.

Many medical writers working in this field are employed by specialist healthcare agencies, whose clients are pharmaceutical companies. In addition, it is important for pharmaceutical companies to have medical writers on their side to validate and critique the work being delivered by the agency medical writers. In particular, it is essential that any outputs in the medical communications field are in line with the relevant regulations. As projects can have an international dimension close liaison with regulatory/legal departments is required to ensure that the regulations for each particular country where the medical communications project will feature are closely followed and adhered to. Medical communications should be focused on the quality of the messages not on the quantity of material being generated. It is also imperative that companies operate in an ethical manner and are transparent in revealing all trial data.

> The role of medical writer calls for attention to detail, good writing skills and team skills.

The role of medical writer calls for attention to detail, good writing skills and team skills. It also requires an analytical mind, an understanding of scientific principles and good English language skills.

The Clinical Study Report

What does a clinical trial report actually consist of?

The clinical study report is the culmination of months or years of data collection and analysis. It brings together the whole process and should provide a comprehensive description of how and why the clinical trial was conducted, what the results were and what they mean. A study report is required for each and every clinical trial, from Phase I to Phase IV. Even trials that are abandoned are written up, albeit in an abbreviated report.

The clinical study report is usually destined to sit as one brick in the building of an application for a license to market a new drug (or device). It does not tell the whole story, but it provides a snapshot of how the drug behaved in a particular group of patients or volunteers.

Eventually, comparisons will be made across studies, therefore, the content and presentation of an individual clinical study report needs to be viewed in the wider context. The messages it gives must reflect the overall aims of the product development program.

The clinical study report essentially follows the pattern of a standard scientific report; it has an introduction, a methods section, a results section, a discussion of the findings and a set of conclusions at the end. It therefore tells a story with a predictable structure. There are international guidelines (produced by the International Conference on Harmonisation; ICH) which provide the structure, in terms of the section headings, subheadings and guidance on the information to include in each section. See Figure 1. These ICH guidelines are not a legal requirement but are universally followed throughout the industry. Some new drugs and devices do not follow the classic development route and therefore the clinical study report may require modifications to its structure. Modifications are permitted by ICH but, even in these cases, writers generally try to follow the ICH structure wherever possible. Following the familiar structure enables the reader to quickly locate particular information.

Study reports range in size, from approximately 50 to 200 pages of text with accompanying tables, figures and listings. A study report has to be factually correct and consistent across all sections. It should be complete, free from ambiguity, well organized and easy to review. It should be written in simple language that is easy to understand and that will not be misinterpreted by readers whose first language is not English. Suitable tables and figures need to be designed and constructed to illustrate particular points; sometimes a well constructed table or figure can convey the message far more quickly than putting all the results in long paragraphs of text.

Figure 1

Clinical Study Report Structure
(from the International Conference on Harmonisation)

1. Title Page
2. Synopsis
3. Table of Contents
4. Ethics
5. Investigators and Study Administrative Structure
6. Introduction
7. Study Objectives
8. Investigational Plan
9. Study Patients
10. Efficacy Evaluation
11. Safety Evaluation
12. Discussion and Overall Conclusions

Figure 1: Clinical Study Report Structure.

In terms of the content, the report should provide a clear explanation of how the study was designed and provide enough information on the methods used so that there is no ambiguity. Although based on the protocol, it may be necessary to clarify methods which were not described in detail in the protocol and the report should also discuss any ways in which the actual methodology was different to that described in the protocol.

The study population is presented in detail in the clinical study report, particularly any differences between the groups or subgroups analyzed. Efficacy and safety results are presented at a number of different levels, from individual patient data to overall summary figures and tables. Finally, the relevance of these results is discussed in relation to the original objectives of the trial and in the context of the whole development program, drawing a few salient conclusions at the end. A synopsis (usually placed at the beginning of the report) provides a summary (2 to 4 pages) of the main features of the trial. This is usually the last part to be written.

How is it assembled?

The authoring team for an individual clinical study report may include as many as 10 people, including representatives from several different departments. Typically there would be representatives from Clinical Monitoring, Medical Affairs, Data Management, Statistics, Drug Safety, and Regulatory Affairs on the authoring team. See Figure 2. Working as part of an authoring team, the medical writer communicates with other team members to obtain information and resolve queries. The medical writer will also chair review meetings at different stages along the process. The writer has to handle the team diplomatically to ensure all the aims and objectives are met and that there is agreement between the whole team on what the key messages are.

> **The writer has to handle the team diplomatically to ensure all the aims and objectives are met...**

Since the medical writer is often responsible for co-ordinating the production of a particular study report and knows what information needs to be included, he/she can be a valuable member of the team throughout the study process. Understanding what the final report will look like enables the medical writer to advise on protocol and case report form (CRF) content. For example, when trying to write up

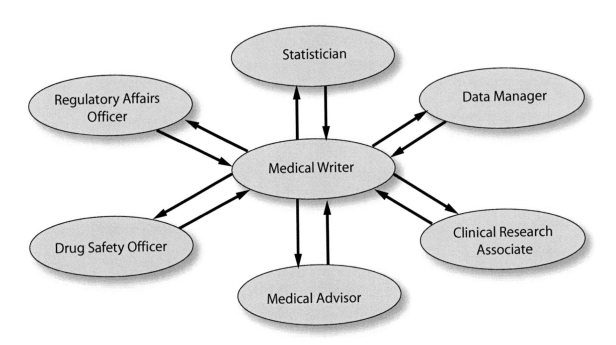

Figure 2: The authoring team.

the study report, it is not going to be possible to comment on the effect of alcohol consumption on blood pressure if there is no space on the CRF for alcohol consumption to be recorded. Medical writers may therefore be asked to review the protocol and CRF for a planned study. In the same way, the medical writer may be asked to review the statistical analysis plan before the analysis is conducted, to see if the proposed tables and listings are going to provide appropriate information for inclusion in the study report.

The clinical study report process is a multi-step process and can involve several drafts. It is unusual for the first draft of a report not to require changes. More usual is that one or two drafts are produced before reaching the final report stage. In some cases, more than two drafts may be required. This may be due to a change in emphasis for a particular product, requiring a different conclusion to be drawn, or it may be due to a tiered system of review where numerous layers of management review the document, each at a different stage. An example of the clinical study report process is shown in Figure 3.

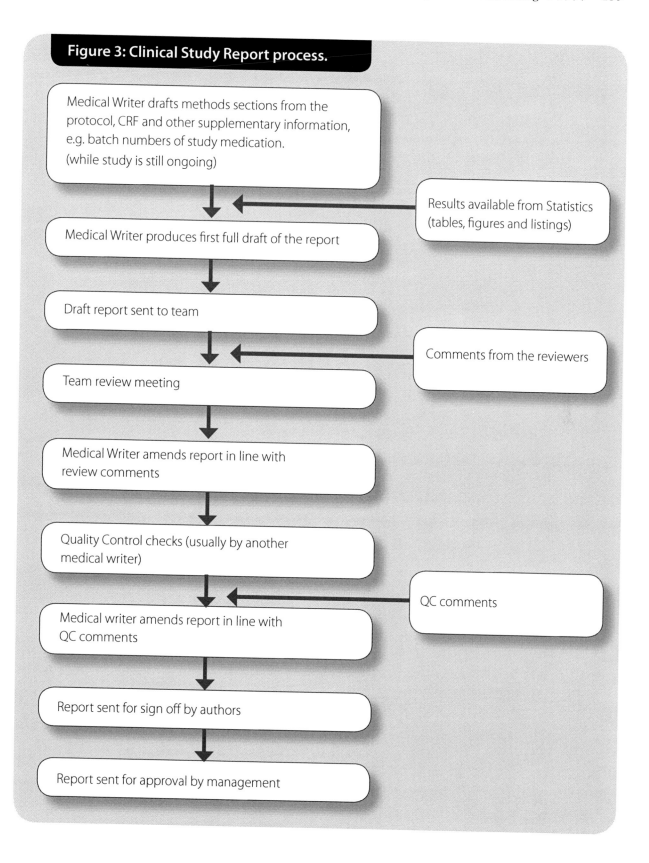

Figure 3: Clinical Study Report process.

Medical Writer drafts methods sections from the protocol, CRF and other supplementary information, e.g. batch numbers of study medication.
(while study is still ongoing)

Results available from Statistics (tables, figures and listings)

Medical Writer produces first full draft of the report

Draft report sent to team

Comments from the reviewers

Team review meeting

Medical Writer amends report in line with review comments

Quality Control checks (usually by another medical writer)

QC comments

Medical writer amends report in line with QC comments

Report sent for sign off by authors

Report sent for approval by management

Other documents

There are a host of other documents associated with clinical trials that need to be written. The principles of clear and accurate communication apply as much to these documents as to the final study report and therefore often fall within the responsibility of Medical Writing. To give a flavor of the variety of documents, here are a few:

The Protocol: Before a clinical trial can even start, the study design and process needs to be clearly, concisely and comprehensively documented in the protocol. Without a well written protocol, the clinical trial is unlikely to get approval from the ethics committee or investigational review board and will at best be delayed and at worse never get off the ground.

The Investigator Brochure: This document is a summary of all the available information on the new drug or device, presented in summary form. It is designed to provide an overview of the pharmacology of the drug, together with results from animal testing and any previous clinical trials. It should contain everything the potential investigator needs to know before starting a clinical trial.

> [T]he major international pharmaceutical associations have a set of agreed, voluntary principles for disclosing information about clinical trials.

Patient information leaflets: These tell the prospective participants what taking part in the clinical trial will involve. It covers things like the number of visits to the clinic, the type of measurements or assessments they will undergo, the nature and duration of the treatment, any precautions they will have to take and their right to withdraw from the trial at any time and for any reason.

Safety reports: If an unexpected, significant adverse event occurs during a clinical trial, a safety report has to be submitted to the regulatory authorities and all participating investigators have to be notified. Each report contains details of the event, and an assessment of the impact on other subjects in this and similar clinical trials.

Publications: Although there are currently no national laws to say that all clinical trials must be published, the legislation may not be far away. At the time of writing, legislation is going through the United States House and Senate which could make publication mandatory; the outcome is awaited. The Declaration of Helsinki states that, "Negative as well as positive results should be published or otherwise made publicly available." The Declaration also states that experimentation not in accordance with its principles should not be accepted for publication. (See Chapter on ethics.)

The pharmaceutical industry is committed to transparency and, as such, the major international pharmaceutical associations have a set of agreed, voluntary principles for disclosing information about clinical trials of marketed products. Guidelines for Good Publication Practice[1] and for the public disclosure of clinical trial results[2] are available, promoting responsible and ethical publication practices.

Data from clinical trials may be published in a journal or presented at scientific meetings as a poster or abstract. The medical writer is often well placed to write an article or poster, particularly if he/she wrote the study report for the data to be published.

The involvement of a professional medical writer in drafting publications can be controversial, especially if the writer is a pharmaceutical company employee. Guidelines have been issued by the European Medical Writers Association[3] which stress the importance of respecting widely recognized authorship criteria and of ensuring that the named authors have full control of the content of the publication. Medical writers also have a professional responsibility to ensure that the papers they write are scientifically valid and are written in accordance with generally accepted ethical standards.

Summary documents

A regulatory submission is organized in a layered fashion. The clinical study reports form one level of a submission, together with non-clinical study reports and quality documentation. Above this level are a series of summary documents. These summary documents bring together results from several studies at once, providing an overview of each area of the development program.

Medical Writers Associations

The two most well known associations of medical writers are the American Medical Writers Association (AMWA) and the European Medical Writers Association (EMWA). AMWA is a much older association, having been in existence since 1940, whereas EMWA began during the early 1990s. There is also an Australasian Medical Writers Association, which was established in 1982. All three associations provide a forum for education, training and professional development.

Each association holds regular meetings and conferences, providing a range of sessions, including keynote speakers, round table discussion and workshops. The main feature of these meetings is the workshop program, designed to provide long-term professional development. Workshop participants receive certification at different levels and in various specialities, by completing a set number of pre-workshop assignments and attending the corresponding workshops. The meetings also provide valuable opportunities for networking and exchanging ideas.

Each association functions independently from the other. However, there are a number of writers who belong to both AMWA and EMWA, providing cross-fertilization of ideas.

> [T]he pharmaceutical market is extremely competitive...

Medical Communications and the Medical Writer

As mentioned earlier, medical writing is also a core part of the medical communications field, with most medical writers employed by specialist healthcare agencies whose clients are pharmaceutical companies. Pharmaceutical companies look for medical communications agencies to develop an appropriate strategy to ensure a favorable launch environment for their product. This means that the appropriate scientific and economic messages must be conveyed to a wide audience. Furthermore, all projects must be vetted by a regulatory/legal expert to ensure that they conform with the regulations of the country where the project will feature. Medical communications has an important influence on current clinical practice but its value depends on how it is used. Therefore a responsible approach by medical writers is paramount.

Medical writers involved in these types of projects must have a thorough understanding of the clinical trials process and how to draw out key scientific messages from clinical data for a diverse range of outputs. Many of these will be influenced by the pharmaceutical company's own goals for the product and so medical writers need to be flexible in order to alter their writing style according to the project in question. Whereas some projects will have a very academic 'feel' to them and will be aimed at a scientific/medical audience, others may have a more commercial slant for a broader audience. Since the pharmaceutical market is extremely competitive, medical writers working in medical communications may also need to keep up to date with the trial results being published on a host of rival products as these may impact on their projects. Commercial projects may involve liasing with marketing departments of pharmaceutical companies, who may have a very different perception of the key messages arising from a clinical trial, and so the medical writer's diplomacy skills will prove essential!

> **The medical writer must understand how to engage with the audience.**

When working in the medical communications field, a medical writer might find him or herself preparing abstracts, manuscripts and reviews for medical journals, medical textbook chapters, slide sets for investigators and company personnel to use at conferences and other events, conference reports, scientific material to be incorporated into material used by marketing departments, internal company physician product guides and perhaps even some patient-focused materials. Frequently, medical writers will find themselves being used on-site for scientific conferences. This involves working in an advisory and editorial capacity to help those presenting clinical trial data at the event. Therefore, in a medical communications role, the medical writer must understand how to engage with the audience, whether they are healthcare professionals, public health authorities or patient organizations.

As mentioned earlier, there has been some controversy about the field of medical communications, with considerable negative media publicity centering around the concept of "ghost writing" for medical journals. Critics state that many of the papers that appear in medical journals cited as having been authored by prominent academics are in fact prepared on their behalf by agency medical writers, who are paid by pharmaceutical companies. Thus the pharmaceutical industry has faced allegations of conveying biased information about its clinical trial data via such papers. Companies have defended this process, detailing the sign-off procedure involving the academics listed, that must be followed from initial drafts of the paper through to the final submission document.

Interestingly, many in the media have called for increasing transparency concerning pharmaceutical industry-sponsored clinical research. Therefore, the use of agency medical writers is seen by the industry and many academics as improving the publication process, since agency medical writers are usually more skilled than trial investigators at summarizing the information in a format that is acceptable to medical journals. Preventing medical writers from being involved in the publication process could exacerbate the problems of non-publication of important clinical trial information. Pharmaceutical companies should use the agency medical writer as an impartial assessor of the strength and accuracy of their trial data and the quality of the messages being produced from it.

> Preventing medical writers from being involved in the publication process could exacerbate the problems of non-publication of important clinical trial information.

In order to respond to the confusion over how findings from industry-sponsored clinical trials are published there are continuing initiatives to standardize the process. These have involved taking into account the viewpoints of industry representatives, academics, investigators and journal editors. Not surprisingly, it has been difficult to achieve consensus. For example, as the pharmaceutical industry is composed of many different organizations, each with their own approach to publications, there is not even a standard industry viewpoint on the ideal system for publishing clinical data.

Many are attempting to follow the approach outlined in the Good Publication Process (GPP) guidelines for pharmaceutical companies[1]. This advises companies to publish the results from all their clinical trials of marketed products and to do so in an accurate, balanced and objective manner[1]. It also urges companies to consult other forms of guidance such as the Uniform Requirements for Manuscripts Submitted to Biomedical Journals developed by the International Committee of Medical Journal Editors (ICMJE)[4] and the

Consolidated Standards of Reporting Trials (CONSORT) statement[5], which consists of a checklist and flow diagram to help improve the quality of reports of randomized controlled trials. Furthermore, many medical writing associations, such as EMWA, have issued their own guidance documents about how professional medical writers should operate when being asked to develop publications on behalf of named authors[3]. Although medical writers should ensure that the publications developed are scientifically valid, the named authors have to take final responsibility for the content of the publication[3].

Summary and conclusions

✦ Medical writing is an integral part of the clinical trial process.

✦ Good clinical research demands effective communication, both to the regulatory authorities and to the wider scientific community. This is the role of the medical writer.

✦ The clinical study report is the culmination of the clinical trial process, providing a comprehensive description of the objectives, methodology, results and conclusions of the trial.

✦ Medical writers are skilled in presenting complex scientific concepts in logical, unambiguous ways.

References

1. Wager E, Field EA, Grossman L. Good publication practice for pharmaceutical companies. Curr Med Res Opin 2003;19(3):149-154.

2. Pharmaceutical Research and Manufacturers of America. Principles on conduct of clinical trials and communication of clinical trial results. www.phrma.org/files/Clinical%20Trials.pdf.

3. Jacobs A, Wagner E. European Medical Writers Association (EMWA) guidelines on the role of medical writers in developing peer-reviewed publications. Curr Med Res Opin 2005;21(2):317-321.

4. ICMJE, Uniform Requirements for Manuscripts Submitted to Biomedical Journals: Writing and Editing for Biomedical Publication. International Committee of Medical Journal Editors, 2006. http://www.icmje.org/icmje.pdf

5. CONSORT, The CONSORT statement. http://www.consort-statement.org/, 2001.

Chapter 12

The clinical trials process: role of the clinical research physician

Dr. Madhu Davies
Consultant in Pharmaceutical Medicine

All clinical trials are unique,
designed to answer a specific
question.

Introduction

It will be clear to those who have read steadily through the book to this point that the conception, planning and execution of a clinical trial is a multi-disciplinary effort involving many different functional roles. Medical staff tend to be a very privileged group in clinical trials management, in that they often have influence at many levels and into various functions as well as providing specific inputs of their own.

Typically, the medic involved in Phase I-III registration studies will be described as a 'clinical research physician' (CRP) and the physician involved with Phase IIIB-IV studies will work in 'Medical Affairs' as their job will typically involve peri-registration and marketing activities. These activities include regulatory and commercial aspects that take place to support the successful registration and launch of the product onto the marketplace. Job titles can be misleading and, particularly in smaller companies, experienced physicians will often fulfill the corporate Medical Director or Chief Medical Officer function, and may be required to span across all Phases of clinical trials (on their own). Similarly, in a larger company, or for those new to clinical research, a single physician may be involved with one study (obviously under supervision). Clinical research physicians may also be employed by Contract Research Organizations (CROs) to whom pharmaceutical companies may delegate the day-to-day management of clinical studies. Clearly in this environment a physician working up to relatively senior levels will retain a very much 'hands on' approach as well as becoming involved in the management activities of the CRO.

The Clinical Research Physician

Where do CRPs come from?

The clinical research physician is typically recruited from clinical practice into industry to be part of a new program and often to be responsible for, under close supervision, a suite of studies, ultimately intended to form part of the registration package. CRP positions will be advertised on company websites, in the medical press and also usually be placed with recruitment consultants.

Typical job advertisement for 'AnyPharm' for a senior Clinical Research Physician to lead a therapy area program:

- Leading the clinical strategy of the Life Cycle Management plan for all [therapy area] products
- Providing advice and guidance to all European affiliates and ensuring strategy is followed
- Ensuring alignment of the various Global teams with the Life Cycle Management Plan
- Responsibility for the scientific design, data interpretation, reporting, publication and messaging of Phase IIIb-IV clinical studies
- You will have significant experience of working in medical affairs and clinical research in the pharmaceutical industry, ideally within the [therapy] area. With proven influencing skills and experience of writing or commissioning publications, you will be suitably medically qualified and have an excellent track record of supporting new and marketed products. In addition, your career to date will include wide-ranging international experience and ideally include time spent in an affiliate organization.

The basic qualifications required are typically eligibility for full registration with the medical board of the country in which the research position is based; adequate clinical experience with a higher post-graduate medical qualification and a clinical specialist or post-graduate degree (Masters, Ph.D., MD/Ph.D.), ideally in a research area relevant to the proposed clinical trial program.

There is often an anxiety among those considering a move from the clinic to industry that they will be perceived by their clinical peers to have 'sold out' or 'gone over to the dark side'. Personally I have found that joining industry has been a fantastic way to retain and grow my medical knowledge. This is possible because industry physicians are at the cutting edge of medicine, and are absolutely expected to be 100% up to speed, so a transfer from the standard clinical / academic route entails losing little and gaining a lot. Many industry physicians also continue to participate in clinics for the first few years of their industry career to keep in touch with their roots.

Maintaining the theme of personal and professional growth and development, there are a number of industry physician associations designed to promote best practice and encourage training education and development. Several universities offer post-graduate training culminating, if successful, in a formal Diploma examination in Pharmaceutical Medicine. In the United Kingdom specific training to become a Specialist in Pharmaceutical Medicine is encouraged.

An established CRP looking for promotion or moving to another company would also be expected to have experience in designing and running clinical trials, prior experience with ethics committees and/or local regulatory activities, relevant experience of collaborating with commercial or marketing groups and ideally, clinical experience in the therapy area as well as undertaking specific training in pharmaceutical medicine alongside the day job.

Whether new to clinical research or experienced, the clinical research physician cannot be successful without excellent interpersonal, influencing and written and verbal communication skills and the ability to cheerfully get on with folk regardless of how difficult things are at the time. This is a very visible role and word soon gets round, both within the company and beyond.

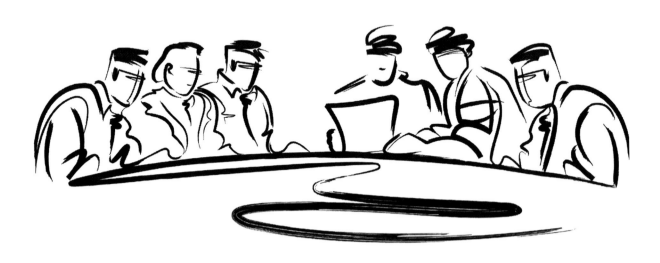

The project team is there to 'keep the show on the road' and management informed appropriately.

Illustration by Wadi Talhami, NY

What do CRPs do? Roles of the Clinical Research Physician

Matrix/project team member

The specifics of what each company expects its clinical research physicians (CRPs) to deliver for them will depend on the nature, size, nationality and geographical spread of that company and also, very importantly, its clinical development philosophy. In particular, does the company run and manage trials in-house or contract the execution and day-to-day management to a CRO with the physician providing 'sponsor oversight' or supervision? Sponsor medical responsibility for the trial is not a 'soft option'! The following are broad roles that CRPs of varying levels of experience would generally be expected to fulfill or develop into with time and experience. They are written from the perspective of a physician working within a sponsoring pharma company but it is not difficult to see which aspects would be covered by the clinical research physician employed by a CRO to run the studies on a day-to-day basis.

In many companies, the CRP will usually be part of a clinical matrix team and project team (please see chapter on project management). The clinical matrix team will typically include representatives from clinical strategy, clinical operations, regulatory affairs, statistics and data management and a medical input as a minimum. Some individuals may have more than one functional role within the team, particularly in the smaller company, where for example, one medic may combine clinical operations including safety, and clinical strategy functions. The project team is usually broader including representatives from all functional areas involved in commercializing a product for example, chemistry, manufacturing and controls (CMC), non-clinical toxicology, regulatory affairs, clinical, safety (in companies where this is a separate group), statistics and data management, commercial and, critically a project manager and /or other senior project leaders. This team is there to 'keep the show on the road' and management informed appropriately of any delays and their anticipated impact on other activities for example, regulatory submissions or commercial activities.

These team-based roles provide a golden opportunity for the physician to contribute broadly across the program using his or her background general medical training and knowledge married with the relevant therapy – area specific input, plus specific medical clinical development inputs as required whilst learning how drug development and indeed, business, works. That's a win-win.

Product development strategy

Depending upon their level of experience, the CRP will be responsible for contributing the medical input to the global development of product strategy either independently or under supervision. This will generally take the form of working with other team members to produce the target product profile of the development candidate (i.e. what you want to be able to say on the data sheet) and the clinical development plan required to support that. Depending on the size of the company, the drafting of the clinical development plan may have inputs from over a dozen people; in a small company it will probably be written by just one or two people-typically the clinical operations director and the medic before being sent on to senior management for review and approval.

Study specific documentation and review

A key element of the CRP's role is their contribution to clinical activities relating to protocol development, efficacy and safety data review, and clinical report writing. Typical areas of input will include the medical rationale for the study, the clinical background and participation in discussion of relevant clinical efficacy and safety endpoints and assessments. This is challenging and fascinating and can be very satisfying to those who enjoy the science of clinical studies.

Medical governance

With appropriate training and experience, the CRP will often be expected to take responsibility for medical governance (i.e., medical/legal and human safety aspects) for individual clinical studies including a medical monitor role and have an excellent understanding of Good Clinical Practice (GCP) and how that will be assured in the current study program. The medical monitor is a physician appointed within the (sponsor) company for each protocol to ensure the responsibilities of the Sponsor, especially with regard to ethics, safety, and the assessment of adverse events are carried out effectively and appropriately.

Some companies split out the safety physician function from that of the Medical Monitor and as this is arguably the most important aspect of a CRP's job, this deserves specific mention here. The safety physician will typically:

✦ maintain awareness of current pharmacovigilance legislation and guidances;

✦ (be part of the) authorization of regulatory authority submission and periodic reports;

✦ generate risk/benefit profiles and risk assessments;

✦ review adverse events and serious adverse events;

✦ assess ongoing risk/benefit; train investigators;

✦ generate regular safety reports for ongoing studies; and

✦ confirm evaluations of causality.

In addition, the safety physician will review major protocol violations for safety implications and consider in consultation with other relevant personnel, what actions will be necessary as a consequence of this.

Clinical operations

The CRP will usually partner with clinical operations to select Investigators and provide support with training and education of these investigators and continuing communication in a formal setting for example, the Investigator's Meeting, or through regular newsletters and study updates. A good relationship with the Investigators is key to ensuring that they remain focused and engaged with the study, as studies are often difficult to do and other competing opportunities may appear more interesting! Additional support to clinical operations will depend on what is needed on a day-to-day basis and what resource is available in the company.

Regulatory support

A very interesting part of the job of the CRP is providing input to the regulatory strategy and responsibility for execution, including involvement in regulatory activities. For example, the Clinical Trial Authorization Application at one end of the development spectrum through to the Marketing Authorization Application at the other. And, of course, the follow up questions on safety and efficacy from the regulatory authorities. This can really challenge the engaged physician who must have a good understanding of the current regulatory environment and regulations per se and provides much scope for broad development. The scope of this support, i.e., local affiliate through to United States, Europe, Japan and Rest of the World will depend on exactly where the CRP sits in the company structure.

Commercial input

An area that really gets most entrepreneurial physicians very excited is the input to their company's commercial needs. This may include input to a regional (United States/Europe/Rest of the World) development plan in order to deliver on the commercial requirements of that region. Together with supporting the approval/launch of pharmaceutical products, this can provide unique development opportunities for the physician. As part of the commercial strategy and development of the product, CRPs will support regional key opinion leader development, advisory board support, publication strategy and other medical activities as required in collaboration with Regional Medical Affairs/Commercial groups. This is often where the earlier Phase CRP, having worked on a program through Phases II and III, finds him or herself transitioning from pure clinical research into the commercial medical affairs arena. This situation may result in an unsuitable fit for the CRP. And while many CRPs are ready for this, enjoy it and thrive, many others will actively seek to work on the earlier development of other products as they miss the clinical research environment.

Management

It may seem odd to include maintaining a high level of current knowledge in the relevant therapeutic area under 'management' but this is retained here as management level physicians will be supervising others. In addition, they will be providing therapeutic and medical guidance, signing off on therapy area development documentation and cannot do so without knowing about the therapy area.

With seniority comes increasing responsibility. This may include responsibility to others on the team who will require people-management, juniors who require mentoring, training and development, and to senior management who will require of the physician the timely execution of key commercial deliverables.

The Medical Advisor

Industry job titles can be very difficult to interpret. What one 'medical advisor' does may not seem to bear much resemblance to the job of another similarly titled individual. From a clinical research perspective, the medical advisor will usually be involved in Phase IIIb-IV activities. These may include activities surrounding the registration period, and developing the product beyond that for extended indications. The actual activities undertaken with regard to this later phase research will be very similar to those described above for the early phases CRP but with a definite emphasis on the commercial value of these clinical trials and how they fit into the marketing mix.

In addition, the medical advisor will have a very 'hands on' approach to medical marketing including the review and approval or marketing materials, input to commercial strategy on a local or regional basis depending on where the advisor sits within the company structure, key opinion leader development and maintenance and a key role in pharmacovigilance. Hence there is significant overlap between this job and that of the 'CRP' – the major difference being the phase of research in which the individuals are involved.

Summary and conclusion

The CRP has a fascinating, privileged and key role in the clinical development and commercialization of medicines. How the individual develops their industry career will depend on their personal preferences, the needs of individual employers and the opportunities available. Whatever the outlook of the individual, life as a CRP offers a real chance to make a difference.

+ The CRP is an integral part of the clinical study team with a range of functional area responsibilities and interactions.
+ Good clinical research demands effective input from each team member. Timely and effective medical input is the role of the CRP.
+ The safety of subjects is paramount. It is the medical monitor's role to assure this.

Suggestions for further reading

The Textbook of Pharmaceutical Medicine, Eds Griffin JP and O'Grady J

BMJ Books/ Blackwell Publishing, Fifth edition 2006

Practice and Principles of Pharmaceutical Medicine, Fletcher AJ, Edwards LD, Fox AW, Stonier P., Wiley and Sons. Second edition. 2007.

Associations:

American Academy of Pharmaceutical Physicians and Investigators (AAPP), www.aapp.org

British Association of Pharmaceutical Physicians (BrAPP), www.brapp.org

International Federation of Associations of Pharmaceutical Physicians (IFAPP), www.ifapp.org

Faculty of Pharmaceutical Medicine of the Royal Colleges of Physicians (UK), www.fpm.org.uk

Chapter 13

Clinical trials and the patient

Ms. Liz Langley, LHA Ltd.

> It is a brave patient who challenges a clinician who they may later rely upon to treat them!

Why does a patient join a clinical trial?

Introduction:

When I was invited to contribute to this excellent book I was initially flattered, and then I realized what a challenging request it actually was. The goal of this book, to help readers new to clinical research understand aspects of the work that is done, is important. My part in this work is to offer thoughts as a patient in a clinical trial.

Clinical trials are not 'clinical' unless they include patients. As a clinical researcher, I found that we could easily overlook the needs, motivations and attitudes of the patient. Such an oversight was done at the researcher's own peril. I worked as a clinical research associate (CRA) in the late 1970s and early 1980s at a time when 'Good Clinical Practice' (GCP) was a new science. Then, informed consent was much less widely used and, indeed, excellent studies were designed with a degree of freedom long gone. Was the patient at the center of all our studies? Of course. But did we always think about the demands we would place upon the patient in sufficient depth? I suspect not. The question today is whether this perception of the patient has that changed and improved?

Studies are devised to prove concepts, to establish efficacy, to investigate effects, to improve practice and to enable new medicines, equipment or techniques to enhance the quality of life for patients. Can we also improve that quality of life or at least self-esteem for those participating in studies?

My background:

- In 1998 I was diagnosed with ductal carcinoma in situ (DCIS) and was offered an elective radical mastectomy with axillary node sampling.
- The surgeon was optimistic that this would be the end of treatment and offered a reconstruction concurrently with the mastectomy.
- I was 42 at the time of diagnosis, with two sons, one of whom was only 3 years of age and both I had breast-fed to 9 months.
- Post-surgery the pathology proved less favorable and I required chemotherapy.
- I agreed to participate in the International Adjuvant Breast Cancer Chemotherapy Randomised Trial, ABC (CT), and Ovarian Ablation or Suppression in Premenopausal Early Breast Cancer Randomised Trial, ABC (OAS).

Entering a clinical trial

First awareness:

As a patient you will have received a diagnosis; often one which you dreaded, sometimes one which has taken you completely by surprise; seldom one you are grateful for. At the end of one consultation or perhaps after many, the subject of a clinical trial may have been mentioned. In my experience if the consulting doctor is one of the investigators it will be discussed with you in an upbeat and positive manner. If they are part of a department undertaking studies but the individual is not directly involved the introduction might be lack luster, and at best presented in a "throw away" manner.

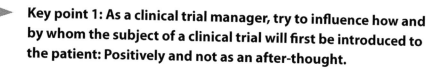 **Key point 1: As a clinical trial manager, try to influence how and by whom the subject of a clinical trial will first be introduced to the patient: Positively and not as an after-thought.**

Key point 2: If you cannot influence the way patients are introduced to the clinical trial, at least know how it is being done. This may explain recruitment and drop-out rate.

Depending on the way in which the topic is raised, the patient's relationship with the individual who mentions it and their general attitude to life at that time (e.g., depression), they may decline to participate or to hear more. In the age of the Internet the patient may have attended a consultation armed to the teeth with in depth knowledge of their condition and the range of clinical trials currently underway investigating new treatment regimens. The consultant may or not react favorably to such knowledge. The interactions in the consulting room are complex and very stressful. It is a brave patient who challenges a clinician who they may later rely upon to treat them!

Key point 3: Wherever possible, present valuable, well prepared information on the study for patient use. Give enough for this to satisfy those who want to know a little and Internet links for those who want more.

So, for those clinical trials managers involved in patient recruitment, the first hurdle to overcome is to ensure that subjects hear about the study in a positive, thorough way. I suspect this relies very heavily upon dedicated and motivated study nurses who hector clinical staff and make sure that potential subjects at least step through the study office door.

Key point 4: Always meet all the team on a study, not just the lead investigator. You need to be able to talk to all the influencers of patient recruitment and answer their questions.

As much as anything, my motivation was my past employment history. I had expected patients to join my studies and now was the time to put up or shut up! There were naturally some other personal and altruist reasons. When I asked several other subjects in my study why they were taking part in the trial, the main reasons were:

♦ Access to the latest therapy

♦ More follow-up than "ordinary" patients

♦ Helping people in the future by increasing medical knowledge, and

♦ I like/trust my doctor.

Access to more follow-up is a major motivation I suspect for patients with oncology diagnoses. The follow-up visits, and the 'fear of the unknown' remain some of the scariest parts of the treatment in the patient's mind. So the chance to see a doctor/nurse more often is a definite plus as you cascade into a long succession of treatment. It is difficult to feel special when told you have a potentially life-threatening condition, you feel cross, very scared, depressed, but certainly not special. Agreeing to become part of clinical trial can actually help a feeling of well-being at a time when that is hard to achieve.

Key point 5: The patient's motivation to participate is important in the decision-making process. Whatever their motivation, it needs to be respected at the time of recruitment. Some want to help others and some want the very best for themselves. It is likely that your study can achieve multiple goals if explained properly.

Initial meeting with study team members

As a patient, you have agreed to attend a briefing meeting on the clinical trial so that you can decide whether or not to participate. The study office is not always the most inspiring room to visit and environment can play a huge part in decisions to join studies. If the office looks a mess with piles of folders, study papers and general signs of disorganization everywhere, I suspect that a number will drop out there and then.

 Key point 6: Access where patient recruitment consultations will take place and try to ensure these are professional but comfortable. If necessary provide lots of storage for report forms etc so that they can be kept tidy!

The study investigators are likely to be asking a patient to participate in new and/or experimental treatment. This is an important and significant decision for the patient. If the team looks haphazard and disorganized, why would I offer them my currently damaged body for experiment? Will they look after that body with care? Or am I just a number? At this delicate stage the patient does not want to be a number or a subject – they are a person and need to matter even for a very short period of time. Patients need to be reassured. They do not want it to be obvious that these briefing sessions have a tight timeframe which must not overrun. Joining a study cannot be a hurried decision because when a patient reflects later why they have joined they need a clear and positive recollection of their immediate motivation.

 Key point 7: Make sure everyone involved in the study "buys" into the study, its goals and anticipated outcomes. This way they will recruit more confident patients who will stay with the protocol.

Explaining complex study protocols to stressed individuals is difficult. The patient is there because they want to say 'yes' but the current challenge of informed consent, the need for detailed explanation of exactly how the study has been designed and what randomization means need to be presented correctly and warmly.

If the study's treatment arm does not look to the patient as though it is a better option, this will become a major stumbling block. If there is a treatment that sounds drastic and is to be done in addition to the already demanding therapy, that too may tax even the most positive of patients. These are huge dilemmas for study designers and the study coordinators who have to recruit patients. Observationally, we need, at the time of design, to be reviewing what exactly we are asking patients to do for the benefit of medical science and think before we commit heroic studies to paper when we might have been able to achieve a similar result by other means.

Key point 7: Is there one, or perhaps a few key goals for the study that can be explained to patients? A goal that they can hold in their heads and perhaps discuss with friends and relations? If there is make sure everyone on the study explains it carefully.

In my particular case, I was well but shocked by the diagnosis. I was not looking forward to six months chemotherapy and I was now about to agree not only to take tamoxifen for five years (or not) but to also have my ovaries ablated/suppressed (or not). The taking of tamoxifen was something I understood was generally well thought of in advanced post-menopausal breast cancer especially for patient with estrogen receptor (ER+) tumors. It was carefully explained to me that the side effects were unpleasant but in many women not debilitating, and that early indications were that there might be survival benefits for those taking tamoxifen. Indeed, this trial was intended to increase the dataset in early premenopausal breast cancer. Additionally ovarian ablation/suppression had been demonstrated to have survival benefits in postmenopausal advanced breast cancer and again this study was to evaluate its use in the younger, less severely affected patient group.

Key point 8: Seek to allay fears with facts and empathy. If the protocol is complex admit it is complex and explain why it is. If treatment will change someone's life, not necessarily for the better, then that will require explanation and the study team will need to have strategies to overcome objections from the patient.

As I sat looking at the study schema, I hoped that I would be randomized to tamoxifen but not to ovarian ablation/suppression. It was somehow the "comfort" of an oral therapy that if I really found impossible I could stop versus the permanent loss of ovaries whose function I suspected were far from defunct. Pregnancy was only three years away from me and now I was facing menopause and yes, I am sorry to say, old age too soon.

Key point 9: Every patient is a vulnerable human and we must consider their feelings at all times even if they don't consider ours.

These fears may sound irrational and ridiculous when matched with the chance of improved survival rates. I had identified these fears to the surgeon as my most important fears at the time of diagnosis because they were highly significant to me. I sat in front of a lovely and empathetic study nurse who I knew wanted me to join the study and I tried to explain to her my fears and concerns. She listened but said that the two treatments needed to be considered together. It was possible that, once I had entered the study, the randomization would offer my preferred combination but that it might not. It was possible just to undertake the tamoxifen part of the study but it was very obvious that the center wanted patients to enter both tamoxifen and ovarian ablation/suppression where possible. She said things like, "well the chemotherapy will probably knock out your ovaries anyway." And although that was true, it did not make the decision any easier. On the positive side, it appeared that each center could use its own preferred practice for the ovaries. It transpired that my center favored suppression with goserelin injections rather than surgical removal. The consolation of this was reduced surgical intervention and the ability to stop suppression if the side effects were too devastating.

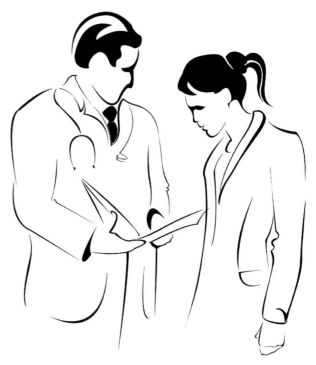

Every patient is a vulnerable human and we must consider their feelings at all times.
Illustration by Wadi Talhami, NY

Second visit and agreement to participate

By now I wanted to take part but I also wanted to feel that it was on my terms. I wanted the study team to understand and acknowledge that I had some misgivings. This comes back to the need for all of us involved in clinical trials to understand how important our subjects are and that they deserve to be treated with empathy. They are not a resource or a set of data. We will expose them to treatments that we know may cause problems and they will largely accept these problems if we treat them individually and well.

 Key point 10: Read the signs of desire, in patients, to participate and build their confidence. Make them aware that you understand their reservations but that their contribution to the overall study means something.

When the randomization came through I was, of course, in the tamoxifen and ovarian ablation/suppression group. The only remaining decision was to be the type of chemotherapy regimen I received. An anthracylin/cyclophosphamide 4 cycle regimen was offered but I chose a CMF (cyclophosphamide, methotrexate, 5-fluorouracil) six cycle bi-monthly regimen because I did not want the excessive susceptibility to simple infections brought home by my three year old!

 Key point 11: Choices empower people. If it is possible for patients to have input into their particular regimen then they are likely to feel more positive about the study.

The study itself

The chemotherapy and tamoxifen were to commence within four weeks of surgery and the ovarian suppression within two months.

I received my first set of quality of life questionnaires direct from The Institute of Cancer Research within four days and then at 3, 6, 9, 18, 30, 48 and 72 months. These were 20 page documents with laborious questionnaires and visual analogue scales for various assessments. There was also a section where patients were encouraged to offer observations and comments. I completed a number of these questionnaires hoping that someone would contact me to perhaps reassure that all was well or ask for more detail. In fact, the only time

I was contacted was when I failed to return the form by the deadline. Then I received a call from the study center reminding me that I was in an important study and that I had agreed to complete it and would I please return the forms as soon as possible.

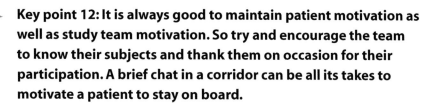 **Key point 12: It is always good to maintain patient motivation as well as study team motivation. So try and encourage the team to know their subjects and thank them on occasion for their participation. A brief chat in a corridor can be all its takes to motivate a patient to stay on board.**

I never saw the study nurse formally again. We passed in the corridor as I came to clinic for chemo. She smiled but was always too busy to speak to me in any depth and the recruiting oncologist really could not understand why I was complaining of troubling menopausal symptoms when I looked so well.

Remarks and conclusion

I now realize that writing this piece has been a valuable, if not cathartic, experience for me. I reflect on the number of studies that I helped design and implement. I believe that I might have designed these and acted differently had I really considered the feelings of those patients I asked to participate. After having been on the other side of the clinical trial, it is much easier to understand why patients default and withdraw.

The treatment I received was exemplary at all stages but it lacked the personal touch – not a mawkish over-sympathetic approach but a positive upbeat gratitude that would have made the whole thing more motivating and uplifting.

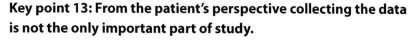 **Key point 13: From the patient's perspective collecting the data is not the only important part of study.**

The final papers were published in Journal of National Cancer Institute Vol 99 Issue 7 April 2007. I know that some clinicians are not sure that they wish to encourage patients to investigate the Internet too much but I think it might be a good piece of PR to inform those who took part that the study has been published, that the results are excellent and to include a brief paragraph of top-line findings. Databases must be good enough to avoid sending information to deceased patients and therefore bereaved relatives. But my observation is that such people often recall the contribution their loved one made and would like to see it noted somewhere.

Key point 14: Consider ways to impart results to patients, where appropriate.

Editorial notes:

Mrs. Liz Langley touched on *Informed Consent* from the patient and human perspective in her section on the initial meeting with the study team members. This initial meeting is part of the process by which the researcher asks the patient's permission to enroll them into a clinical trial. In order for the patient to be adequately informed this meeting must provide clear and unambiguous information on the aim of the study, what it is trying to establish, what the treatments are, what the patient needs to do, and the possible risks and benefits. This information is supplemented by an information sheet. When the patient has had sufficient time to think things through and ask questions, an informed consent form is signed. The critical importance of informed consent in studies conducted to 'good clinical practices' (GCP) standards has been noted by the references in the chapter on study monitoring. There are a few very exceptional circumstances in which a patient can be enrolled into a study without giving their consent. An example would be a study in unconscious head injury patients BUT consent must be obtained from a relative or other legal representative and careful safeguards will have been put in place to protect any patients entering these studies as part of the ethical review process.

Liz did not use patient support groups but she comments that these may be useful for some individuals. Readers for whom this is relevant may choose to look up possible support groups on the Internet. They can also ask at the unit where they receive their treatment.

Additional resource:

The United Kingdom Clinical Research Collaboration publishes some informative booklets on clinical trials aimed and patients and careers. http://www.ukcrc.org/publications/informationbooklets.aspx

Chapter 14

The future
of clinical trials

Dr. Faiz Kermani

> It is the 'human factor' that really makes a clinical trial a success.

The future of clinical trials

Read just about any newspaper and you will likely come across one report or another citing preliminary findings of laboratory-based scientific research as if they represent an absolute, guaranteed breakthrough in treating a particular disease. Although there is no doubt that many of these findings are of great importance, the only way of building on the promise of pharmaceutical discovery research and verifying its potential is by conducting clinical trials. As such, clinical trials continue to represent the vital step in developing medicines. Furthermore, it is often forgotten that the data generated in clinical trials has implications for how successful the medicine will be viewed in the long term when ranked against newer medicines.

The contributions to this book have shown that an understanding of clinical trials is essential for those involved in the development of new medicines and for those interested in participating as patients. It is impossible to cover all the factors that might influence the future of clinical trials, but a few are explored in this chapter.

Most major trials are conducted on a commercial basis and pharmaceutical and biotech companies must plan ahead in order to fund the various stages of clinical research necessary before a drug ever reaches the market. In this respect, financial factors will have a major influence on the future of clinical trials. However, promising a new drug or therapy might be, only those with adequate financial resources will be able to embark on the clinical trials necessary for the drug to reach the market and yet retain the flexibility to run additional studies, if so required, once a drug has been launched on the market.

> [A]n understanding of clinical trials is essential for those involved in the development of new medicines and for those interested in participating as patients.

When investing in clinical trials, it is important to understand that drug development is a risky venture and that many of the promising candidates being tested *will* fail and that a range of factors may be responsible. Therefore, companies must have enough funding to account for these failures and must also have systems in place that can identify potential failures early on and eliminate them from progressing to the more costly stages of clinical trials. Even now there are examples of companies that been unprepared for trial setbacks and have been driven out of business.

Every year, pharmaceutical and biotech companies spend an increasing amount of money on R&D, but the proportion that needs to be allocated to clinical trials also continues to grow. A 2002 survey of US pharmaceutical companies found that the inflation-adjusted increases in clinical R&D costs were more than five times greater than the costs for preclinical work.[1] This is certainly not a new problem, and many companies frequently experience a heavy increase in expenditure when their compounds reach clinical trials.

One way that pharmaceutical companies deal with this financial pressure has been to outsource the clinical trial work to specialized contract research organizations (CROs). According to the Tufts Center for the Study of Drug Development, since 2001, spending by pharmaceutical companies on outsourced clinical research services has grown nearly 16% annually, exceeding the 11% rate for overall spending on development.[2] CROs can conduct clinical trials for pharmaceutical sponsors at a lower cost. This can permit the pharmaceutical company to concentrate their in-house efforts on other parts of the R&D process.

Pharmaceutical companies have been conducting a growing number of clinical trials in so-called emerging markets.

Outsourcing also allows pharmaceutical companies to keep their staffing to a minimum as CRO staff take on the day-to-day tasks for the trial, which require considerable numbers of staff. This approach particularly benefits smaller companies, who have limited resources. All the signs are that most clinical trials in the future will feature some involvement of CROs. As a result, the CRO sector is booming and many clinical researchers have found such organizations to represent an exciting career option, due to the variety of clinical trials they become exposed to.

Another reaction to the financial pressures has been to expand clinical trial work overseas. Pharmaceutical companies have been conducting a growing number of clinical trials in so-called emerging markets. The major drug development regions of the world remain North America, Europe and Japan, but markets such as those in Asia, Latin America and Africa have emerged as important locations for clinical trials being run by pharmaceutical and biotech companies [Figure 1]. Clinical trial costs in emerging regions are frequently less than in the main pharmaceutical markets, due to fast patient recruitment and lower

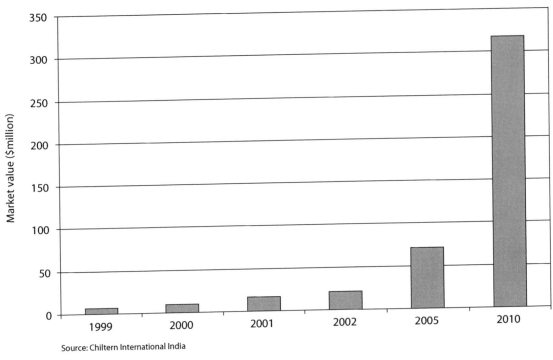

Source: Chiltern International India

Figure 1: Growth of the Indian Clinical Trials Market.

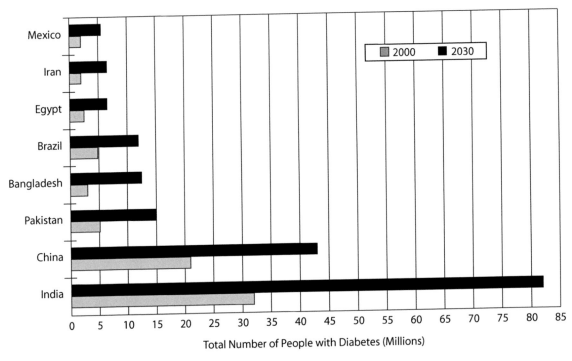

Sources: World Health Organization

Figure 2: Diabetes estimates and projections in Selected Emerging Countries.

operating costs. Furthermore, these regions often feature a sizeable group of patients with the therapeutic conditions that pharmaceutical companies are interested in [Figure 2]. As a result there is growing competition between pharmaceutical companies to recruit patients for their trials in these regions.

The trend in using emerging regions has further significance since they are also becoming important markets for new medicines. Through clinical trials, local physicians gain experience of new products and therefore it is in a company's interests to base some clinical research in these locations. In fact in some countries, regulators expect to see some local clinical development of a product to have taken place.

However, the move to working in emerging markets has also led to additional pressures for the pharmaceutical industry. In particular, since some patients are unable to afford modern medicines there have been demands that the pharmaceutical industry continue to provide them with access to medicines after completion of the trial. Frequently, emerging regions are not a market for the drug being developed and thus when the clinical trials for a product are successful these patients may never again have access to the product.

As regulatory agencies demand an increasing level of information on the drugs being tested, technology has become an invaluable part of the clinical trial process. The range of clinical trial technology solutions available continues to grow and pharmaceutical companies are often faced with difficult choices in knowing which particular technology will really benefit their clinical study projects. However, many companies understand that they will need to invest in these new approaches if they are to increase their chances of success. As many technologies can automate processes, they often improve the quality of the clinical trial data generated, and speed up the overall time taken to conduct studies.

Although advances in technology will benefit drug development projects, it is the 'human factor' that really makes a clinical trial a success. This shows no signs of changing in the future. As has been emphasized in the chapters so far, clinical trials involve staff who are specialized in a variety of different disciplines, but it is not good enough to simply have people who have been well trained in their own individual fields. Effective communication between these different staff, each of whom will bring a unique professional viewpoint, is essential when making important project decisions. It is no coincidence that the job market for clinical trials is fiercely competitive, with companies eager to hire talented individuals with expertise in the various clinical trial disciplines. Similarly, training has become of vital importance so that staff can remain up-to-date with the standards expected for the conduct of clinical trials.

As many clinical trials are international, those running such projects must also understand the regulations and the ethical considerations in the different countries where trial centers will be based.

In order to predict the future it is important to understand the past and learn from previous mistakes. Modern clinical trials are international projects involving huge financial investment, specialist technology, and the management of staff with expertise in a range of disciplines. This can lead to a highly pressurized environment for those working on such projects, with all attention focused on ensuring that the various stages envisaged for the trial are efficiently conducted. When meeting the expectations of senior management, it is important for clinical trial professionals to retain an objective viewpoint about the trial being conducted and ensure that project commitments do not interfere with moral and legal responsibilities.

An exciting influence on future clinical trials will be pharmacogenomics

History shows us that results are not all that matters in a clinical trial and that certain clinical trial professionals have not always behaved with integrity when dealing with patients. Fortunately, regulatory mechanisms and staff training have improved and continue to help shape the evolution of clinical trials so that past errors and oversights are not repeated. Aside from following legal guidelines, clinical trials personnel should take it upon themselves to ensure that they always safeguard the rights of patients and treat them with dignity and respect. Many patients have a great interest in the finer details of the clinical trials in which they participate and are eager to learn more about new medicines [Figure 3], but clinical trial professionals often overlook this. Since better public understanding of clinical trials will benefit the pharmaceutical industry when recruiting participants in the future, clinical trial professionals could do more to engage with such individuals. Recent initiatives by the pharmaceutical industry to provide more information on which clinical trials they are conducting are to be welcomed. These initiatives allow patients to feel part of

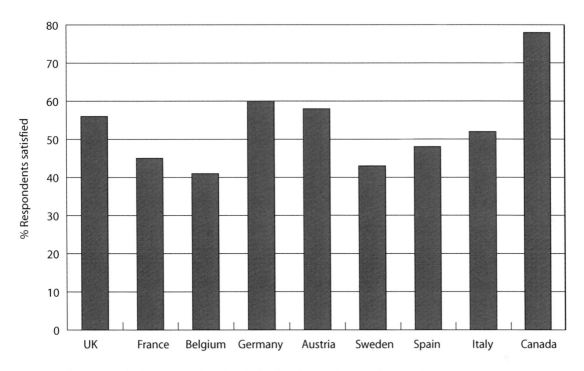

Source: International Alliance of Patients' Organizations (http://www.patientsorganizations.org)

Figure 3: Patient satisfaction with ability to access information on new medicines or treatments.

a process that generates medical advances that will benefit the population as a whole.

An exciting influence on future clinical trials will be pharmacogenomics, as it is now well accepted that a significant proportion of differential drug response is genetic in origin. This genetic angle has often not been fully appreciated, but new developments are driving the use of this information in clinical trials. Pharmacogenomics uses genetic analysis to identify potential targets for medicines or to identify large-scale differences in the patterns of gene expression in response to chemical compounds.[3] Supporters of pharmacogenomics believe that it will revolutionize clinical trials [Figure 4] and improve their success, as more will be known about the compounds being tested in relation to the genetic make-up of participants. In this scenario, pharmaceutical companies could exclude subjects, for whom a particular drug would be harmful or ineffective. By screening patients who would be appropriate for the drug being tested in the trial, considerable resources and time may be saved.

Phase I – drug metabolism genes based on pre-clinical data	Reduce risk by checking whether drug will cause problems in genetic sub-groups
Phase II – drug metabolism genes from phase I and activity genes from drug discovery	Increase confidence by associating weak response with genotype
Phase III – significant SNPs* from phase I + II. Additional testing to explain rare adverse events and non-responders	Reduce cost by using genotyping to increase efficacy thereby reducing trial size

Source: DxS (www.dxsgenotyping.com

Single nucleotide polymorphisms or SNPs are DNA sequence variations that occur when a single nucleotide in the genome sequence is altered. Since variations in DNA sequence can have a major impact on how humans respond to disease SNPs are of great interest for researchers.
Source: What are SNPs? Genome Projects of the US Department of Energy Office of Science
http://www.ornl.gov/sci/techresources/Human_Genome/faq/snps.shtml

Figure 4: Pharmacogenomics and clinical trials.

Despite the inevitability of pharmacogenomics affecting clinical trials, so far it has only had a modest impact at best. This is because many pharmaceutical companies have been very successful in developing drugs that can be used by a variety of patients and there is a fear that pharmacogenomics will segment markets and drastically reduce revenues.[4] Given that it costs pharmaceutical companies a tremendous amount of money to develop a new drug, will they be willing to invest in the R&D process if the end product is only considered applicable to a small portion of the population? Another worry of pharmaceutical companies is that they are still unclear about what pharmacogenomic information regulatory agencies are seeking for their test products. However, this situation is changing, with the FDA appearing to be the regulatory leader in this respect.[4] The FDA is developing detailed guidance documents that provide information on its current thinking and the use of pharmacogenomics for regulatory decision making. It has also introduced a genomics training program for its staff and is collaborating with foreign regulatory agencies to develop international guidelines.

References

1. Anon. Industry Profile 2002. The Pharmaceutical Research and Manufacturers of America (PhRMA) (2002). http://www.phrma.org

2. Getz K and Wenger J High times for the CRO heavyweights. Partnerships with CROs and other Outsourcing Partners. March 2007 Official Magazine (2007). http://www.cropartners.com

3. Pharmacogenetics and Personalised Medicine – Key Facts. http://www.dxsgenotyping.com

4. Kermani F. Pharmacogenomics. Pharmaceutical Physician 2007;17(4):8-11

Glossary

ABC (CT) and ABC (OAS) Trials	Adjuvant Breast Cancer Chemotherapy Randomised Trial and Ovarian Ablation or Suppression in Premenopausal Early Breast Cancer Randomized Trial
ADME	Absorption, distribution, metabolism and excretion
Ae (0-t)	Amount (of drug) excreted in urine between time zero and stated time
AIDS	Acquired ImmunoDeficiency Syndrome
AMA	American Medical Association
AMWA	American Medical Writers Association
ANDA	Abbreviated New Drug Application
API	Active pharmaceutical ingredient
AUC	Area under the curve
AUC	Area under the concentration-time curve
B (e.g. $100B)	Billion
BLA	Biologic License Application
CBER	Center for Biologics Evaluation and Research
CDER	Center for Drug Evaluation and Research
CEO	Chief Executive Officer
CFR	Code of Federal Regulations
CLr	Renal clearance
cm	Centimeters
Cmax	Maximum concentration
CMC	Chemistry, manufacturing and controls
CMF	Cyclophosphamide, methotrexate, 5-fluorouracil
CNS	Central nervous system
CONSORT	Consolidated Standards of Reporting Trials
COX	Cyclooxygenase
CRA	Clinical research associate
CRF	Case record or report form
CRO	Contract research organisation
CRP	Clinical Research Physician
CTA	Clinical Trial Application
CTD	Common Technical Document
CTMS	Clinical trial management systems
CYP	Cytochrome
DCSI	Ductal carcinoma in situ

DESI	Drug Efficacy Study Implementation
DHHS	Department of Health and Human Services
EC	Ethics Committee
ECG	Electrocardiogram
eCRF	Electronic Case Report Forms
EDC	Electronic data capture
EDC	Electronic data capture
EMEA	European Medicines Agency
EMWA	European Medical Writers Association
EPOS	Electronic point of sales
ePRO	Electronic reported patient outcomes
ER	Estrogen receptor
EU	European Union
Eur Ph	European Pharmacopoeia
FDA	Food and Drug Administration
Fe	Fraction(of dose) excreted in the urine
FIH	First in human
FIM	First in man
GCP	"Good Clinical Practice"
HbA1c	Glycosylated haemoglobin A1c
HLGT	High level group term
HLT	High level term
ICH	International Council on Harmonisation (of Technical Requirements for Registration of Pharmaceuticals for Human Use)
ICMJE	International Committee of Medical Journal Editors
IFPMA	International Federation of Pharmaceutical Manufacturers and Associations
IMPD	Investigational Medicinal Product Dossier
IND	Investigational New Drug (Application)
IRB	Institutional Review Board
ISSE	Integrated summary of safety and efficacy
IVR	Interactive voice response (systems)
IWR	Interactive web response
JAMA	Journal of the American Medical association
JP	Japanese Pharmacopoeia
KPM	Key performance measure
LLT	Lower level term

M (e.g. $100M)	Million
MD	Master's degree (also used in the USA to mean Medical Doctor)
MedDRA	Medical Dictionary for Regulatory Affairs
NDA	New Drug Application
NIH	National Institutes of Health
NSAID	Non steroidal anti-inflammatory drug
OPHRP	Office of Human Research Protections
OPRR, now OHRP	Office of Protection from Research Risks
Patient (subject)	Patient with illness under study participating in a clinical trial, usually Phases I-IV
PC	Personal computer
PhD	Doctor of Philosophy
PK	Pharmacokinetic
POC	Proof of concept
PR	Public relations
PT	Preferred term
R & D	Research and Development
RIVM	Rijksinstituut voor Volksgezondheid en Milieu (National Institute for Public Health and the Environment)
SACHRP	Secretary's Advisory Committee for Human Research Protections
SAE	Serious adverse event
SAP	Statistical analysis plan
SD	Standard deviation
SMO	Site maintenance organisation
SOC	System organ class
Subject	Participant in a clinical trial. Term often reserved for healthy subjects (i.e. healthy individuals participating in Phase I clinical research.
Tmax	Time to maximum concentration
TNF	Tumour Necrosis factor
TPP	Target product profile
US(A)	United States of America
USP	United States Pharmacopoeia
USPHS	U.S. Public Health Service
WMA	World Medical Association
WWII	World War II